SOUP RECIPES COOKBOOK

Heavenly Tasty Soup Recipes With Simple Instructions

(A Collection of Delicious Soup Recipes)

Kimberly Burton

Published by Alex Howard

© **Kimberly Burton**

All Rights Reserved

Soup Recipes Cookbook: Heavenly Tasty Soup Recipes With Simple Instructions (A Collection of Delicious Soup Recipes)

ISBN 978-1-990169-37-3

All rights reserved. No part of this guide may be reproduced in any form without permission in writing from the publisher except in the case of brief quotations embodied in critical articles or reviews.

Legal & Disclaimer

The information contained in this book is not designed to replace or take the place of any form of medicine or professional medical advice. The information in this book has been provided for educational and entertainment purposes only.

The information contained in this book has been compiled from sources deemed reliable, and it is accurate to the best of the Author's knowledge; however, the Author cannot guarantee its accuracy and validity and cannot be held liable for any errors or omissions. Changes are periodically made to this book. You must consult your doctor or get professional medical advice before using any of the suggested remedies, techniques, or information in this book.

Table of contents

PART 1 1

INTRODUCTION 2

BACON & BEEF STEW 3

ONION, KALE, CHICKPEA, AND CHICKEN SOUP 6

SOULFUL CHICKEN SOUP 8

CREAMY LEEK AND PARSNIP SOUP 10

SMOKY HAM AND SPLIT PEA SOUP 12

POTATO SOUP 14

CHICKEN AND CORNBREAD DUMPLING 17

BLACK GARLIC AND LENTIL SOUP 20

SMOKED SAUSAGE CASSOULET 23

SLOW COOKER CIOPPINO 25

SUGAR BABY BUTTERNUT SOUP 28

SHREDDED CHICKEN TORTILLA SOUP 30

CREAMY WHITE BEAN SOUP WITH SMOKED HAM HOCKS 32

TORTILLA SOUP 34

SEAFOOD GUMBO 36

TOMATO-RED PEPPER GAZPACHO WITH FRESH VEGETABLE MEDLEY 40

TURKEY ANDOUILLE SAUSAGE GUMBO 43

EASY BRUNSWICK STEW 45

EASY CHICKEN AND DUMPLINGS 47

COCONUT-CURRY CHICKEN SOUP 49

CLASSIC CHICKEN SOUP 52

HEARTY CHICKEN SOUP 54

AVOCADO-BUTTERMILK SOUP WITH CRAB SALAD 56

Italian Wedding Risotto Soup	58
Avocado Gazpacho With Sourdough Croutons	60
Carrot Soup With Parmesan Crisps	62
White Bean And Chorizo Soup	64
Two-Bean Soup With Tomato-Chive Crostini	66
Golden Gazpacho	68
Simple Cream Of Broccoli Soup	70
Creamy Garlic Soup	72
Caribbean Black Bean Soup	74
Vegetable-Beef Soup	76
Garden Minestrone	78
Bacon-Corn Chowder With Shrimp	81
French Onion Soup	83
Cheesy Potato Soup	85
Slow Cooker Chicken, Bacon, And Potato Soup	87
Slow Cooker Chicken Chili	90
White Bean Soup	93
Italian Wedding Soup	95
Farmhouse Chicken Chowder	97
Lentil And KumQuat Soup	100
Red Lentil Soup	102
Potlikker Soup	104
Carrot-Ginger Soup	106
Gingery Lentil Soup	108
Hearty Minestrone Soup	110
Provencal Fish Soup	113
Chicken-Vegetable Soup	116
Smoky Shrimp And Chicken Gumbo	118
Corn Relish	122

BBQ Chicken Soup 124

Hearty Zucchini Soup 126

South-Of-The-Border Beef Stew 128

Arugula Soup 130

Colombian Chicken Soup 132

Chilled Avocado And Yogurt Soup 135

Mexican Chicken Soup 137

Cucumber Gazpacho With Toasted Rye Croutons 139

Southwest Seafood Chowder 141

Lemon Grass Chicken Soup 144

Andouille, Crab And Oyster Gumbo 147

Southwestern Chicken Soup 150

Avgolemono Chicken Soup With Rice 152

Wild Rice And Mushroom Soup With Chicken 154

Carrot Soup With Brown Butter, Pecans, And Yogurt 156

Chard And White Bean Soup 159

Baked Potato And Bacon Soup 161

Amish Chicken Soup 163

CONCLUSION 165

PART 2 166

Fish Chowder 167

Cream Of Black Carrots With Spinach Pesto And Toasted Pine Nuts 169

Lentil Soup 171

Shrimp Bisque 173

Lentil Soup With Sausage 175

Cream Of Spinach Soup 177

Split Pea Soup With Ham 179

Egg Flower Soup 181

Tortilla Soup 183
Pork Ramen 185
Minestrone 187
Potato Wakame Miso Soup 189
Black Bean Soup 191

Part 1

Introduction

An excellent recipe yields a great dish. But the recipe is not the only factor that affects the integrity of a subsequent dish. A lot of other factors like the flavorful leftover pot roast, a bumper crop of fresh zucchini and an aromatic bunch of basil, are part of what make any slow-simmered ingredients a justly unique, inspiring chef-d'oeuvre. Anthropologists argued a lot about the origin of the first ever pot of soup. Some believe that it started with the Neanderthals who softened their foods in water in a hollowed piece of bark. Others even talk about the new evidence of European and African tribes learning to cook plants and meat together in animals' sealed stomach cavities, as well as South Americans using hollowed turtle shells as their containers for stew and soup. Meanwhile, purists assert that the first real stews and soups began around 10,000 B.C. when ceramic pots were used in South America where peppers were added to chilies. Stews and soups were referenced in the oldest surviving cookbooks such as those dating to the 3rd century. In the middle Ages, chicken soup was used to treat diseases. Ancient American accounts of food attribute the origins of recipes and soup traditions to the French, German, and English influences. Native American influences were also evident, particularly their use of wild greens and tree nuts. History recorded from the colonial period clearly shows that through the years, soup has been regarded as a dish that fostered a sense of community, which involved sharing and generosity among members. During the Great Depression, soup became everyone's lifesaver. Nourishment and Satisfaction are the major reasons why people of today valued these dishes the way our forefathers did. Eating soups is a suitable way of sharing great times with loved ones. There are varieties of soup all over the world, so this book is centered to help us in experiencing other cultures through their cuisines flavors, and improving our culinary knowledge and skillsets.

Bacon & Beef Stew

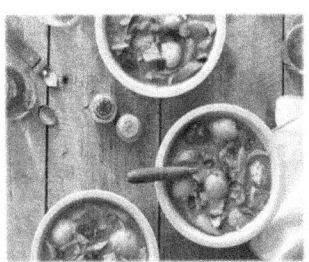

Rich bacon and beef paired perfectly with beer, mustard, and red wine vinegar will create a complex well-rounded flavor profile. This recipe comes together to makes 16 cups which is enough for 12 generous servings. Be sure to use a low heat setting sodium beef broth in order to maintain the balanced of salt level. You can serve it with cornbread, crusty bread, or butter rolls.

ACTIVE TIME: **30 mins**

TOTAL TIME: **1 hour**

YIELD: 12 - servings

SERVING SIZE: (about 1 1/3 cups)

Bacon & Beef Stew

Ingredients

8 ounces' of bacon (about 7-8 slices),

Chopped 4 medium carrots, cut into ½ -in. pieces (about 2 ½ cups)

1 large red onion (about 10 oz.), cut into ½ -in. pieces

Chopped 4 garlic cloves, of about 2 Tbsp.

1 cup beer

¼ cup of all-purpose flour

8 cups of low heat setting-sodium beef broth

1 teaspoon of kosher salt

½ teaspoon of black pepper

12 ounces of baby golden potatoes

1 ½ pounds of Perfect Roasted Beef Softloin

3 tablespoons of coarse-grain mustard

1 teaspoon of red wine vinegar

½ cup of chopped fresh flat-leaf parsley

Preparation

1. Cook the bacon in a large Dutch oven over medium-high heat setting until crisp, for about 8 minutes.
2. Transfer the bacon to a plate lined with paper towels, while reserving 2 tablespoons of drippings in Dutch oven.
3. Add the carrots and onion to the drippings in the Dutch oven then cook and stir often, until it beginnings to soften, for about 4 to 6 minutes.
4. Add garlic then cook and stir it occasionally for 1 minute.
5. Add beer and cook about 5 minutes, then stir and scrap in order to loosen the browned bits from bottom of the Dutch oven.

6. Constantly Stir the and cook the flour until the mixture is thickened and beginning to brown.
7. Mix in broth, salt, and pepper constantly.
8. Reduce the heat to medium-low heat setting, and add the potatoes then cover and cook for about 20 minutes when the potatoes will get soft.
9. Stir the Beef, mustard, vinegar, and cooked bacon.
10. Sprinkle with parsley, and serve immediately.

Onion, Kale, Chickpea, And Chicken Soup

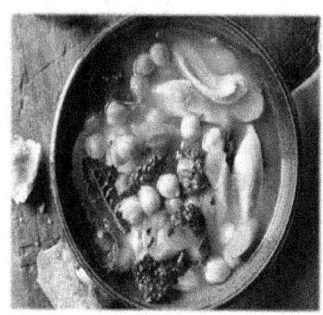

Few things beat a steaming bowl of veggie-packed chicken soup on a crisp autumn evening, and this one happens to be a perfect potion for the seasonal chills. You can leave the thyme sprigs in the broth . Serve around them, so that they will keep releasing the herbaceous goodness into any leftovers.

YIELD: 4 - servings

SERVING SIZE: (about 1 ½ cups)

Onions, Kale, Chickpea, And Chicken Soup

Ingredients

1 teaspoon of olive oil

1 cup of pre-chopped onion

½ cup of diagonally cut carrot

½ teaspoon of crushed red pepper

3/8 teaspoon of kosher salt

3 crushed garlic cloves,

2 thyme sprigs

4 cups of unsalted chicken stock

1 (15-ounce) can of rinsed and drained unsalted chickpeas,

2 cups of chopped Lacinato kale

4 ounces of shredded skinless, boneless rotisserie chicken thigh heat setting

4 ounces of shredded skinless, boneless rotisserie chicken breast

1 teaspoon of low heater-sodium soy sauce

Preparation
1. Heat a large saucepan over medium-high heat setting level of heat.
2. Add the oil swirl to coat.
3. Add the onion and the next 5 ingredients through thyme and cook for 3 minutes and stir it occasionally.
4. Add the stock and chickpeas to pan and cook.
5. Add the kale and chicken to pan then reduce heat, and cook for 5 minutes.
6. Add and stir the soy sauce and discard thyme sprigs.

Soulful Chicken Soup

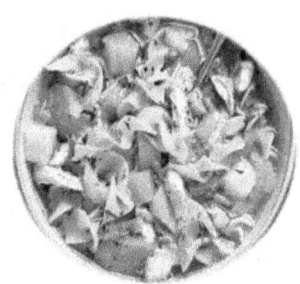

No dish is quite as soothing as a hearty bowl of chicken noodle soup. Slow cookers couldn't have made the road to comfort any easier. Simply toss in the ingredients, switch on, and then walk away. We love old-fashioned, wide egg noodles for this recipe. To make sure they aren't mushy and overcooked, don't leave them in the slow cooker any longer than 10 minutes.

HANDS ON TIME: **20 mins**

TOTAL TIME: 8 hour 20 mins

YIELD: Make 11 cups

Soulful Chicken Soup

Ingredients

2 pounds of skinned and trimmed bone-in chicken thigh,

3 medium carrots, cut into ½ -inch pieces (1 ¼ cups)

1 celery root, cut into ½ -inch pieces (2 cups)

1 medium cleaned and chopped leek, white and light green parts only,

2 peeled and smashed garlic cloves

2 fresh of thyme sprigs

2 fresh of sage sprigs

1 fresh of rosemary sprig

1 bay leaf

1 ½ teaspoons of table salt

1 teaspoon of fresh grinded black pepper

8 cups of chicken broth

2 cups of wide egg noodles

3 tablespoons of finely chopped fresh parsley

1 teaspoon of fresh lemon juice

Preparation
1. Place the chicken and the next 11 ingredients into a 6-qt. slow cooker.
2. Cover and cook on low heat setting for 6 hours or until the chicken and the vegetables are soft and chicken separated from its bone.
3. Remove the chicken from slow cooker.
4. Dice the meat, and discard bones.
5. Return the meat to slow cooker.
6. Add the noodles thyme then cover and cook on high heat setting for about 15 to 20 minutes or until noodles are soft.
7. Add the lemon juice.
8. Serve immediately, and garnish with any leftover chopped fresh parsley.

Creamy Leek And Parsnip Soup

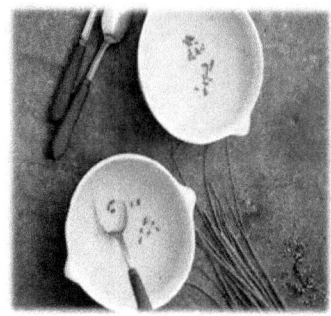

This delicious Creamy Leek and Parsnip Soup is perfect for serving on a chilly fall evening.

HANDS ON TIME: **15 mins**

TOTAL TIME: **55 mins**

YIELD: 4 servings

Creamy Leek and Parsnip Soup

Ingredients

2 tablespoons of unsalted butter

3 leeks, trimmed, halved lengthwise, cut crosswise into ½ -inch-thick slices

5 thinly sliced medium parsnips (about 1 lb.),

Salt and pepper

4 ½ cups of LOW heat setting-sodium chicken broth

½ cup of heavy cream

1 teaspoon of snipped chives

Preparation
1. Melt the butter in a large heavy saucepan over medium heat setting.
2. Add leeks, parsnips, ½ tsp. of salt and ¼ tsp. pepper.
3. Cook and stir often, until it softens but not browned for about 10 minutes.
4. Pour in 4 cups of broth, and increase heat to high heat setting then bring to a full boil.
5. Reduce the heat to medium-low heat setting and cook while partially covered, stir occasionally, until the vegetables are very soft, for about 30 minutes.
6. Let it get cold slightly.
7. Blend the soup in a blender and blend
8. Return soup to saucepan and add cream.
9. Warm over low heat setting and season well with salt and pepper.
10. Thin with remaining broth if the soup is too thick.
11. Serve it into a warmed soup bowls, garnish it with a pinch of chives, and serve.

Smoky Ham And Split Pea Soup

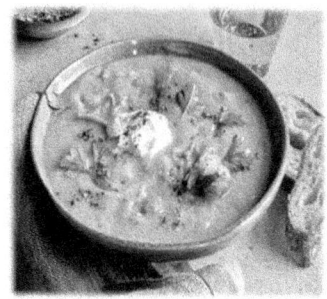

Potatoes contribute starchiness and silky thickness, while sweet carrots and salty ham balance out the peas' light, earthy flavor. Leftovers fare well in the freezer, so say hello to your new favorite make-ahead soup. Garnish with parsley and additional pepper, if desired.

HANDS ON TIME: **15 mins**

TOTAL TIME: 8 hour 15 mins

YIELD: 8 servings

SERVING SIZE: (about 1 ¼ cups)

Smoky Ham and Split Pea Soup

Ingredients

1 pound of rinsed and drained dried green split peas

1 ½ cups of cubed peeled Yukon gold potatoes

5 chopped garlic cloves,

1 cup of chopped onion

1 cup of chopped celery

1 cup of chopped peeled carrot

1 large bay leaf

1 teaspoon of freshly grinded black pepper

¾ teaspoon of kosher salt

2 pounds of smoked ham hocks

6 cups of water

½ cup of light sour cream

Preparation

1) Layer the peas and the next 9 ingredients (through ham) in the order listed in a 6-quart electric slow cooker.
2) Gently pour 6 cups of water over the top.
3) Cover and cook on low heat setting for 8 hours.
4) Remove the ham hocks from slow cooker.
5) Remove the meat from bones, and cut it into bite-sized pieces and discard skin and bones.
6) Discard the bay leaf.
7) Coarsely mash the soup to the desired consistency, and add additional hot water to make it thin, if desired.
8) Add the chopped ham.
9) Divide the soup evenly among 8 bowls and top each serving with 1 teaspoon of sour cream.

Potato Soup

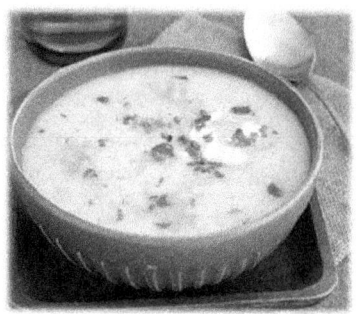

This classic potato soup recipe is warm, comforting, and so delicious. It is an ultimate bowl of comfort food. Because more cheese is always better, this classic soup gets a double hit of cheese, both stirred into the soup and sprinkled over the top. Bacon bits lend a baked potato flavor and feel to this creamy, crowd-pleasing soup. Simply place the ingredients into a slow cooker and let it do all of the work for you.

HANDS ON TIME: **15 mins**

YIELD: 8 servings

SERVING SIZE: (about about 1 cup of soup, 1 teaspoon of sour cream, 1 ½ teaspoons of cheese, 1 teaspoon of bacon, and ½ teaspoon of chives)

Potato Soup

Ingredients

3 bacon slices

1 cup chopped of onion

3 pounds of baking potatoes, peeled and cut into ¼ -inch-thick slices

Cooking spray

½ cup of water

2 (14.5-ounce) CANs of fat-free, low heater-sodium chicken broth

½ of teaspoon of salt

½ of teaspoon of freshly grinded black pepper

2 cups of 1% low heat setting-fat milk

4 ounces of divided shredded reduced-fat sharp cheddar cheese (about 1 cup)

½ cup of light sour cream

4 teaspoons of chopped fresh chives

Preparation
1. Cook the bacon in a large nonstick skillet over medium heat setting until it is crisp.
2. Remove the bacon from pan, while reserving 2 teaspoons of drippings in pan crumble bacon.
3. Add onion to the drippings and cook for 3 minutes or until soft.
4. Place potato slices and onion in a 5-quart electric slow cooker coated with cooking spray.
5. Add ½ cup of water and the next 3 ingredients (through pepper) and stir.
6. Cover and cook on low heat setting for 8 hours or until potatoes are soft.

7. Mash the mixture with a potato masher and add milk and ¾ cup of cheese.
8. Increase the heat to his RA.
9. Cover and cook on high heat seting for 20 minutes or until mixture is thoroughly heated.
10. Serve the soup into bowls and top with sour cream and remaining ¼ cup cheese then sprinkle with bacon and chives.

Chicken And Cornbread Dumpling

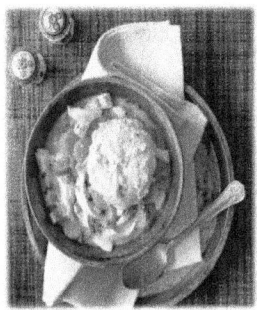

Make a classic chicken and dumplings recipe even more Southern by topping the vegetable-and-chicken-packed stew with cornbread dumplings.

HANDS ON TIME: **30 mins**

TOTAL TIME: 5 hours 40 mins

YIELD: 8 servings

Chicken and Cornbread Dumpling

Ingredients

3 bacon slices

1 cup chopped of onion

3 pounds of baking potatoes, peeled and cut into ¼ -inch-thick slices

Cooking spray

½ cup of water

2 (14.5-ounce) cans of fat-free, low heater-sodium chicken broth

½ of teaspoon of salt

½ of teaspoon of freshly grinded black pepper

2 cups of 1% low heat setting-fat milk

4 ounces of divided shredded reduced-fat sharp cheddar cheese (about 1 cup)

½ cup of light sour cream

4 teaspoons of chopped fresh chives

Preparation
1. Rub the chicken pieces with salt, pepper, and poultry seasoning.
2. Place the breasts in a 6-qt. slow cooker and top with thigh.
3. Add the carrots and the next 3 ingredients.
4. Mix the soup and broth together until it gets smooth.
5. Pour the soup mixture over vegetables.
6. Cover and cook on high heat setting for 3 ½ hours or until the chicken shreds easily with a fork.
7. Remove the chicken and let it cool for 10 minutes.
8. Bone and shred the chicken.
9. Stir the chicken into a soup-and-vegetable mixture.
10. Cover and cook on high heat setting for 1 hour or until boiling.
11. Mix the flour and the next 3 ingredients together.
12. Make a well in center of mixture.
13. Add the milk, butter, thyme, and parsley to dry the ingredients, gently stir until moistened.
14. Drop dough by ¼ cupful into the cooking chicken mixture, leaving about ¼ -inch space between the dumplings.

15. Cover and cook on high heat setting for 30 to 35 minutes or until the dumplings are doubled in size.

Black Garlic And Lentil Soup

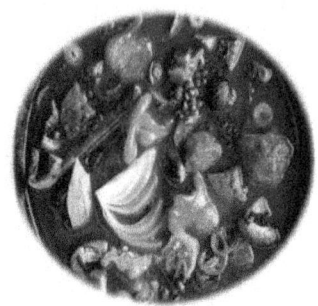

This earthy soup is best with Dried chilies, paprika sausage, hot paprika, and black garlic--regular garlic roasted for days until it turns sweet and jet black, with a licorice-like flavor which gives the soup a rounded spiciness.

TOTAL TIME: 1 hour 30 mins

YIELD: Serves 6 to 8 (about 14 cups)

Black Garlic and Lentil Soup

Ingredients

1 teaspoon of lard or grapeseed oil

1 white onion, cut into half-moons ¼ -in. thick

2 green stemmed and seeded bell peppers, and cut into ½ -in. dice

1 serrano stemmed Chili, halved lengthwise, and cut into thin half-moons

6 cups of Bar Tartine Chicken Broth or divided store-bought reduced-sodium chicken broth

25 peeled Black Garlic cloves, home-made or store-bought, or roasted regular garlic

8 dried arbol chilies or 1 tbsp. of red pepper flakes

3 ripe medium-size cored and roughly chopped tomatoes

4 cups of Sprouted Black Lentils or 1 ¾ cups of regular dried black lentils

12 ounces of dry-cured paprika sausage, such as Hungarian gyulai or Spanish chorizo, or pepperoni

12 finely chopped garlic cloves,

12 ounces' of sliced thin button mushrooms,

2 bay leaves

1 to 2 tbsp. of hot Hungarian paprika

2 tablespoons of apple cider vinegar

2 teaspoons of kosher salt

Black pepper

1 cup of roasted red peppers, cut into 1-in. chunks

Sour cream, chopped green onions, and chopped fresh cilantro, for topping

Preparation
1. Heat a large cast-iron frying pan over medium-high heat setting until a drop of water flicked on the surface sizzles.
2. Melt the lard in a pan and add onion, bell peppers, and serrano.
3. Cook, and stir occasionally, until vegetables are well charred on the edges but not blackened for about 15 minutes.

4. Let it cool, then chop coarsely.
5. Mix 2 cups of broth, the black garlic, and arbol chilies in a blender,
6. Purée until smooth.
7. Cut the sausage into quarters lengthwise, then thickly crosswise.
8. Put it in a large pot and add the black garlic purée, and the remaining 4 cups of broth, tomatoes, lentils, garlic, mushrooms, and bay leaves.
9. Make if cook over medium heat setting, while covered but do not let boil.
10. Add the paprika, peppers, and charred vegetables and cook gently, covered, until the lentils begin to fall apart and make the soup thick for about 20 minutes more.
11. Discard bay leaves.
12. Add vinegar and salt, and season with black pepper.
13. Serve soup into bowls and top each of them with sour cream, green onions, and cilantro.

Smoked Sausage Cassoulet

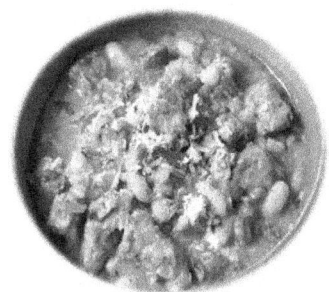

This hearty soup is exploding with flavors. Meat lovers will crave this bacon-packed and sausage-enriched delight. For a thicker consistency, let the cassouwait 30 minutes before serving.

YIELD: 8 servings (serving size: 1 cup of cassoulet, 1 of teaspoon of cheese, and 1 of teaspoon of parsley)

Smoked Sausage Cassoulet

Ingredients

2 bacon slices

2 cups of chopped onion

1 teaspoon of dried thyme

½ teaspoon of dried rosemary

3 minced garlic cloves

½ of teaspoon of salt

½ teaspoon of freshly grinded black pepper

2 (14.5-ounce) cans of drained diced tomatoes

2 (15-ounce) cans of Great Northern rinsed and drained beans,

1-pound of trimmed lean boneless pork loin roast, cut into 1-inch cubes

½ pound of reduced-fat smoked sausage, cut into ½-inch cubes

8 teaspoons of finely shredded fresh Parmesan cheese

8 teaspoons of chopped fresh flat-leaf parsley

Preparation
1. Cook the bacon in a large skillet over medium-high heat setting until crisp.
2. Remove the bacon from pan and crumble.
3. Add onion, thyme, rosemary, and garlic to drippings in the pan and cook for 3 minutes or until soft.
4. Stir the crumbled bacon, salt, pepper, and tomatoes and boil.
5. Reduce the Heat and place half of beans in a large bowl, mash with a potato masher until it is chunky.
6. Add the remaining half of beans, pork, and sausage and stir well.
7. Place half of bean the mixture in a 3 ½-quart electric slow cooker top with half of tomato mixture.
8. Repeat layers, then cover and cook on low heat setting for 5 hours.
9. Serve into bowls and sprinkle with Parmesan cheese and parsley.

Slow Cooker Cioppino

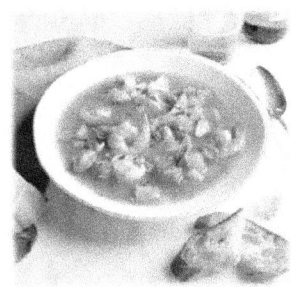

Cooking the base of this rich stew in the slow cooker allows the ultimate flavor concentration. When you're almost ready to serve, add raw fish to poach quickly. A signature dish of the West Coast, cioppino can be made with a wide variety of fish and shellfish, so feel free to experiment with your favorites.

HANDS ON TIME: **20 mins**

TOTAL TIME: 7 hour 45 mins

YIELD: Serves 4 (serving size: 2 cups)

Slow Cooker Cioppino

Ingredients

2 tablespoons of extra-virgin olive oil

1 ½ cups of chopped onion

1 ½ cups of chopped fennel bulb

10 sliced garlic cloves

1 cup of dry white wine

2 teaspoons of tomato paste

½ of cup water

2 tablespoons of chopped fresh oregano

2 tablespoons of chopped fresh thyme

¾ teaspoon of crushed red pepper

3/8 teaspoon of kosher salt

½ pound of chopped fresh tomatoes

2 (2-inch) lemon rind strips

2 bay leaves

1 (26-ounce) box of chopped tomatoes

¾ pound of cod, cut into 2-inch pieces

½ pound of sea scallops

½ pound of peeled and deveined medium shrimp

1 teaspoon of fresh lemon juice

¼ cup of fresh basil leaves

Preparation
1. Heat a large skillet over medium-high heat setting.
2. Add oil swirl to coat.
3. Add onion, fennel, and garlic to pan and cook for 3 minutes or until soft.
4. Add wine and tomato paste to pan, and stir well then boil.
5. Cook for 2 minutes, and stir occasionally.
6. Carefully pour the onion mixture into a 6-quart electric slow cooker.
7. Add ½ cup water and the next 8 ingredients (through boxed tomatoes) to a slow cooker.
8. Then cover and cook on low heat setting for 7 hours.
9. Uncover and discard lemon rind and bay leaves.

10. Add cod, scallops, shrimp, and lemon juice.
11. Cover and cook on low heat setting for about 13 to 15 minutes or until fish flakes easily when tested with a fork.
12. Garnish with fresh basil.

Sugar Baby Butternut Soup

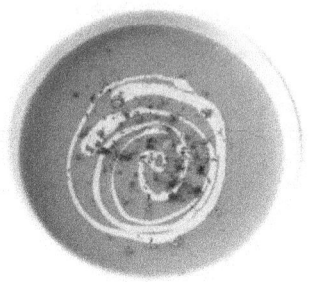

This great autumnal soup gets a dose of added warmth, sweetness, depth from Sugar Babies, a classic Candy that is comprised of caramelized sugar and buttery flavor notes. If you find yourself with leftover Halloween Candy, put it to good use as a surprising ingredient in this fantastic soup. While most would probably opt to use leftover Candy in a dessert, this soup takes creativity to the next level by incorporating it into a savory dish. Grab a spoonful and dig right in!

HANDS ON TIME: 10 mins

TOTAL TIME: 30 mins

YIELD: Serves 6 (serving size: 1 cup each)

Sugar Baby Butternut Soup

Ingredients

2 tablespoons of unsalted butter

1 ½ cups of chopped onion

2 teaspoons of minced garlic

6 cups of cubed butternut squash

2 cups of vegetable stock

¼ cup of Sugar Babies Candy

1 ½ of teaspoons of kosher salt

1 cup of heavy cream

½ cup of sour cream

1 ½ teaspoon of fresh thyme leaves

¾ teaspoon of paprika

Preparation
1. Melt the butter in a Dutch oven over medium low heat setting.
2. Add the onion and garlic to the pan and stir often while cooking, until onions are slightly browned, for about 10 minutes.
3. dd the squash, stock, Sugar Babies, and salt, then boil over high heat Setting.
4. Reduce heat to medium low heat setting, cover, and cook until the squash is soft, for about 15 minutes.
5. Blend the soup in a food processor until it is smooth.
6. Return soup to the Dutch oven and add cream then cook over medium-low heat setting until it is a warmed al-through
7. Divide the soup evenly among 6 serving bowls.
8. Top the servings evenly with sour cream, thyme, and paprika.

Shredded Chicken Tortilla Soup

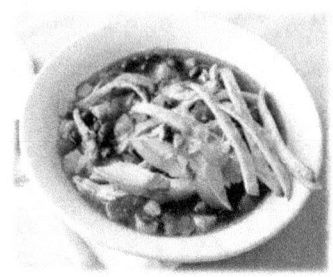

Use Chicken and Mushroom Stroganoff ingredients to prepare this tortilla soup topped with homemade tortilla strips, avocado, cilantro, and lime wedges.

YIELD: Serves 6 (serving size: 1 cup each)

Shredded Chicken Tortilla Soup

Ingredients

1 (6-inch) corn tortilla

Cooking spray

5 teaspoons of Canola oil

1 ½ cups of chopped zucchini

1 cup of chopped onion

¼ cup of chopped cilantro

1 teaspoon of chopped jalapeño

1/8 teaspoon of kosher salt

2 minced garlic cloves

2 bay leaves

1 ½ tablespoons of chili powder

1 teaspoon of grinded cumin

4 cups of reserved stock from Chicken and Mushroom Stroganoff

1 (14.5-ounce) CAN of unsalted fire-roasted diced tomatoes

¾ cup Canned unsalted black beans

½ teaspoon of kosher salt

8 ounces reserved chicken breast and dark meat from Chicken and Mushroom Stroganoff

½ cup of sliced avocado

½ cup of cilantro

4 lime wedges

Preparation
1. Cut tortilla into ½-inch strips and coat with cooking spray.
2. Bake at 375° for 10 minutes.
3. Heat the Canola oil in a large Dutch oven over medium heat setting.
4. Add zucchini, onion, ¼ cup of chopped cilantro, jalapeño, 1/8 teaspoon of kosher salt, minced garlic, and bay leaves and cook for 7 minutes.
5. Add the chili powder and cumin.
6. Add stock and diced tomatoes, then boil.
7. Add black beans, ½ teaspoon of kosher salt, and chicken breast and dark meat and cook for 5 minutes.
8. Remove and discard the bay leaves.
9. Divide among 4 bowls and top with tortilla strips, avocado, ½ cup cilantro, and lime wedges.

Creamy White Bean Soup With Smoked Ham Hocks

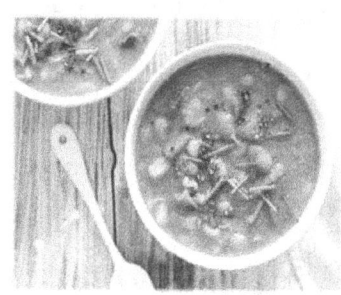

Creamy, starchy, and filling, this hearty, rustic soup is the epitome of comfort. And convenient: Beans go in dry - no need to soak.

HANDS ON TIME: 10 mins

TOTAL TIME: 8 hours 10 mins

YIELD: Serves 8 (serving size: about 1 cup)

Creamy White Bean Soup with Smoked Ham Hocks

Ingredients

2 tablespoons of olive oil

1 ½ cups of chopped onion

1 cup of diced celery

1 cup of diced carrot

1 teaspoon of chopped fresh thyme

6 chopped garlic cloves,

2 pounds of smoked ham hocks

1 pound of dried Great Northern beans

2 (26-ounce) containers of unsalted chicken stock

¼ cup of minced fresh chives

1 teaspoon of freshly grinded black pepper

Preparation
1. Heat a skillet over medium-high heat setting.
2. Add oil to the pan and swirl to coat.
3. Add onion and the next 4 ingredients (through garlic) then cook for 10 minutes or until vegetables are soft.
4. Scrape the onion mixture into a 6-quart electric slow cooker.
5. Add hocks, beans, and stock.
6. Cover and cook on low heat setting for 8 hours or overnight.
7. Remove the hocks from pan and let it cool slightly.
8. Remove the meat from bones and discard the fat, skin, and bones.
9. Chop the meat and add the beans then cook for 10 minutes to allow the flavors to mix.
10. Sprinkle with chives and black pepper.

Tortilla Soup

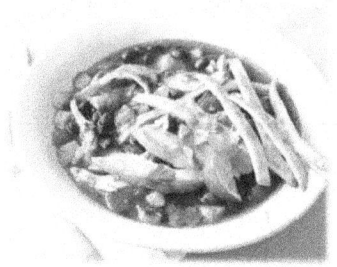

Soup and the slow cooker are natural combos, and this recipe for Tortilla Soup doesn't disappoint.

HANDS ON TIME: 10 mins

TOTAL TIME: 7 hours 10 mins

YIELD: About 10 cups

Tortilla Soup

Ingredients

1 ¾ pound of skinned and boned chicken thigh

1 (12-oz.) bag of frozen and thawed whole kernel yellow corn

1 large chopped onion

2 pressed garlic cloves

2 (14-oz.) cans of reduced-sodium fat-free chicken broth

1 (14-oz.) can of tomato blend

1 (10-oz.) can of diced tomatoes and green chilies

1 teaspoon of smoked paprika

2 teaspoons of grinded cumin

1 teaspoon of chili powder

1 bay leaf

4 (5 ½ -inch) corn tortillas

Toppings: fresh cilantro, shredded Cheddar cheese, sliced jalapeños and avocados

Preparation
1. Add the first 11 ingredients in a 4-qt. slow cooker.
2. Cover and cook on high heat setting 7 to 8 hours.
3. Discard bay leaf and shred chicken.
4. Preheat the oven to 375°.
5. Cut tortillas into ¼ -inch-wide strips, and place it on a baking sheet.
6. Bake it at 375° for 5 minutes.
7. Stir and bake for 5 more minutes or until crisp.
8. Add the table salt to make it tasty.
9. Serve soup with tortilla strips and toppings.

Seafood Gumbo

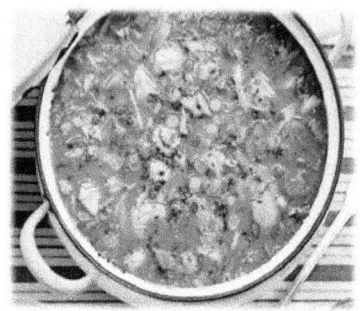

The genius of this menu is that most of the work can be done ahead of time.

HANDS ON TIME: 1 hour 35 mins

TOTAL TIME: 2 hours 25 mins

YIELD: About 5 quarts

Seafood Gumbo

Ingredients

1-pound of fresh lump crabmeat

3 pounds 'of medium-size raw shrimp (with heads)

Pinch of kosher salt

6 tablespoons of divided oil

2 pounds of thawed and frozen sliced okra,

½ teaspoon of kosher salt

1-pound of thinly sliced andouille sausage

2 tablespoons of all-purpose flour

2 cups of finely chopped yellow onion

1 cup of finely chopped celery

1 cup of finely chopped green bell pepper

4 minced garlic cloves

1 cup of divided chopped green onions

1 (6-oz.) of can tomato paste

3 bay leaves

1 teaspoon of finely chopped fresh thyme

2 teaspoons of kosher salt

1 teaspoon of hot sauce

¼ teaspoon of grinded red pepper

½ teaspoon of grinded black pepper

1 teaspoon of Worcestershire sauce

1 (14.5-oz.) can of drained and coarsely chopped, liquid reserved tomatoes,

1 pt. of oysters (between 2 dozen and 3 dozen)

¼ cup of finely chopped fresh flat-leaf parsley

Hot cooked long-grain rice

Preparation

1. Pick the crabmeat, and remove every bits of shell
2. Remove the shrimp shells and heads.
3. Cover and refrigerate shrimp, and place shells and heads in a large stockpot.
4. Add 8 cups of water and a generous pinch of salt, and boil over high heat Setting.
5. Reduce the heat to medium-low heat setting, and cook, while partially covered, for 1 hour.

6. Let it cool down for 30 minutes, then pour the stock through a fine wire-mesh strainer, and reserve for use.
7. Discard shells and heads.
8. Heat 2 Tbsp. of oil in a large heavy skillet over medium heat setting, and add okra. Sprinkle with ½ tsp. salt, and cook for 10 minutes.
9. Set it aside the okra, and wipe out the skillet.
10. Heat another teaspoon of oil in the skillet over Medium-high heat setting, and cook the andouille for about 8 minutes or until brown.
11. Heat the remaining 3 Tbsp. of oil in a large heavy pot over high heat Setting.
12. Add the flour and reduce heat to medium, then cook and stir it constantly for about 10 minutes or until roux turns medium-to-dark brown.
13. Add the yellow onions, celery, and bell pepper, and cook for 4 to 5 minutes or until vegetables begin to soften.
14. Add garlic and ½ cup of green onions, and cook for 3 more minutes.
15. Add the tomato paste and the next 7 ingredients.
16. Add the tomatoes and 1/3 cup of their liquid and gradually add the shrimp stock.
17. Add the reserved sausage and okra, then cover and boil over high heat Setting.
18. Reduce the heat to medium-low heat setting, and cook for 30 minutes.
19. Add the shrimp and the remaining green onions, and cook for 3 minutes.
20. Add the crabmeat, oysters, and parsley, and cook for 1 minute.
21. Reduce the Heat then taste and add salt, if desired.

22. Serve over rice.

Tomato-Red Pepper Gazpacho With Fresh Vegetable Medley

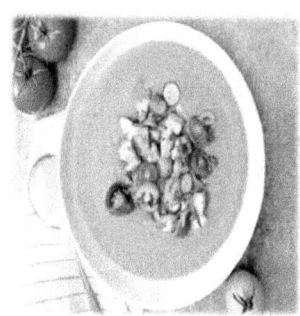

Topping tomato and red pepper-flavored gazpacho with fresh veggies makes a refreshing summer soup.

HANDS ON TIME: 50 mins

TOTAL TIME: 2 hours 50 mins

YIELD: Makes 4 servings

Tomato-Red Pepper Gazpacho with Fresh Vegetable Medley

Ingredients

2 divided red bell peppers,

5 large ripe tomatoes (about 2 pounds)

2 cups of chopped peeled English cucumber

½ cup chopped of green onion

3 tablespoons of extra-virgin olive oil

2 tablespoons of white wine vinegar

1 ½ teaspoons of kosher salt

½ teaspoon of freshly grinded black pepper

1 smashed large garlic clove

Fresh Vegetable Medley

Garnish: fresh flat-leaf parsley leaves

Preparation
1. Preheat broiler to high heat setting.
2. Cut the bell peppers in half lengthwise and discard seeds and membranes.
3. Place the pepper halves and cut sides down, on an aluminum foil-lined baking sheet, flattening the peppers with the palm of your hand.
4. Boil for 10 minutes or until peppers are blackened.
5. Remove the pan from the oven, and wrap the peppers in the aluminum foil.
6. Wait for 10 minutes, peel and dice 2 tablespoons of roasted peppers, and set it aside (for Fresh Vegetable Medley) then place the remaining roasted red peppers in a blender.
7. Bring a large saucepan of water to a boil.
8. Score 5 tomatoes, and score the bottoms in an X shape with the tip of a paring knife.
9. Add the tomatoes to boiling water and boil for 1 minute.
10. Drain and plunge the tomatoes into ice water.
11. And wait for 3 minutes.
12. Peel and coarsely chop tomatoes then discard the skins
13. Add the chopped tomatoes, cucumber, and the next 6 ingredients to blender and process until it is smooth.
14. Pour the mixture into a bowl and cover while it chills for at least 2 hours.

15. Divide gazpacho evenly among 4 soup bowls, and top with Fresh Vegetable Medley.
16. Add the Garnish, if desired.

Turkey Andouille Sausage Gumbo

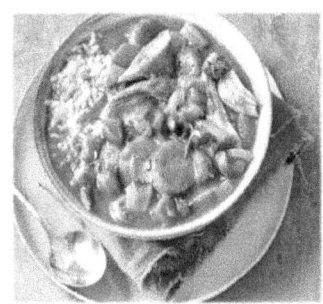

Topping tomato and red pepper-flavored gazpacho with fresh This gumbo is a great use for leftover roasted turkey, though cooked chicken will also work. We skip the long-stirred roux here in favor of filé powder, a thickener made from the sassafras plant look for it on the spice aisle. For the best results, add the filé powder off the heat.

HANDS ON TIME: 30 mins

TOTAL TIME: 55 mins

YIELD: Serves 8 (serving size: about 1 cup of gumbo and ½ cup rice)

Turkey andouille Sausage Gumbo

Ingredients

2 center-cut of chopped bacon slices

¾ cup of chopped onion

½ cup of chopped green bell pepper

½ cup of chopped celery

2 large minced garlic cloves,

4 cups of unsalted chicken stock

½ cup of chopped yellow bell pepper

¾ teaspoon of kosher salt

6 ounces' of thinly sliced andouille sausage links,

1 (14.5-ounce) can of undrained and unsalted diced tomatoes

1 (10-ounce) package of sliced frozen okra

¼ cup chopped of fresh flat-leaf parsley

2 teaspoons of chopped fresh thyme

9 ounces of shredded cooked skinless, boneless turkey breast, (1 ½ cups)

2 teaspoons of filé powder

4 cups of hot cooked rice

Preparation
1. Cook the bacon in a large Dutch oven over medium heat setting for 4 minutes or until crisp.
2. Remove bacon from pan with a slotted spoon.
3. Add the onion, green bell pepper, celery, and garlic to the drippings in the pan then for cook 5 minutes.
4. Add the stock, yellow bell pepper, salt, sausage, tomatoes, and okra to the pan then boil.
5. Reduce the heat, and cook 20 minutes.
6. Add the parsley, thyme, and turkey and cook for 2 minutes or until it is thoroughly heated.
7. Remove the pan from heat and add the filé powder.
8. Divide rice among 8 bowl and top evenly with gumbo.
9. Sprinkle evenly with the reserved bacon.

Easy Brunswick Stew

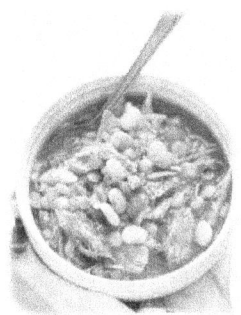

Cooking on low heat setting for a long time makes the meat extremely soft, so it shreds easily high heat Setting yields a less soft product.

PREP TIME: 15 mins

TOTAL TIME: 55 mins

YIELD: 8 - servings

Easy Brunswick Stew

Ingredients

3 pounds of boneless pork shoulder roast

3 medium-size of new peeled and chopped potatoes

1 large chopped onion,

1 (28-ounce) can of crushed tomatoes

1 (18-ounce) bottle of barbecue sauce

1 (14-ounce) can of chicken broth

1 (9-ounce) package of frozen and thawed baby lima beans,

1 (9-ounce) package of thawed and frozen corn,

6 tablespoons of brown sugar

1 teaspoon of salt

Preparation
1. Trim, roast and cut the pork into 2-inch pieces.
2. Stir all ingredients in a 6-quart slow cooker together.
3. Cover and cook on low heat setting 10 to 12 hours or until potatoes are fork-soft.
4. Remove the pork with a slotted spoon, and shred.
5. Return shredded pork to slow cooker, and stir well.
6. Serve stew into bowls.

Easy Chicken And Dumplings

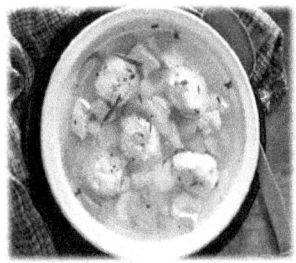

Pillow heat settingy dumplings flecked with fragrant fresh herbs cook drop-style in the stock mixture.

PREP TIME: 20 mins

TOTAL TIME: 40 mins

YIELD: Serves 4 (serving size: 1 ½ cups of soup and 4 dumplings)

Easy Chicken and Dumplings

Ingredients

1 teaspoon of olive oil

2 tablespoons of divided chopped fresh thyme,

2 tablespoons of divided chopped fresh tarragon,

2 celery stalks, cut diagonally into ¼ -inch-thick slices

2 carrots, cut diagonally into ¼ -inch-thick slices

1 chopped medium onion

2 minced garlic cloves

3 cups of unsalted chicken stock

- 1 pound of skinless, boneless chicken breast halves, cut into ¾-inch pieces
- ¼ teaspoon of kosher salt, divided
- ½ teaspoon of freshly divided and grinded black pepper
- 4.5 ounces of all-purpose flour
- 1 teaspoon of baking powder
- 2 tablespoons of butter
- ½ cup of 2% reduced-fat milk

Preparation
1. Heat a large Dutch oven over medium-high heat setting.
2. Add oil to pan and add 1 teaspoon of thyme, 1 tablespoon of tarragon, celery, carrot, onion, and garlic and cook for 5 minutes or until vegetables are crisp-soft.
3. Add the stock and then boil.
4. Add the chicken, 1/8 teaspoons of salt, and ¼ teaspoon of pepper.
5. Reduce the heat to medium, cover it and cook for 10 minutes or until the chicken is done.
6. Add the flour, baking powder, remaining 1 teaspoon of thyme, remaining 1 tablespoon of tarragon, remaining 1/8 teaspoons of salt, and remaining ¼ teaspoon of pepper in a bowl.
7. Cut in butter with a pastry blender or 2 knives until mixture resembles coarse meal.
8. Add the milk stir until it is moist.
9. Drop 2 teaspoons of dough, into the stock mixture, in order to form 16 dumplings.
10. Cover and cook for 7 minutes or until the dumplings are cooked through.

Coconut-Curry Chicken Soup

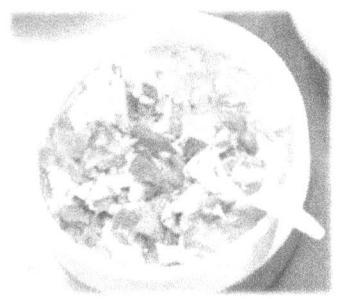

Snow peas, spinach, and chicken breast give this 5-star Coconut-Curry Chicken Soup flavor, texture, and a wealth of nutrients.

PREP TIME: 20 mins

TOTAL TIME: 40 mins

YIELD: 7 servings (serving size: 2 cups of soup and 1 lime wedge)

Coconut-Curry Chicken Soup

Ingredients

4 cups of water

3 cups of fresh spinach leaves

½ pound of trimmed snow peas, cut in half crosswise

1 (5 ¾-ounce) package of pad Thai noodles (wide rice stick noodles)

1 teaspoon of Canola oil

¼ cup of thinly sliced shallots

2 teaspoons of red curry paste

1 ½ teaspoons of curry powder

½ teaspoon of grinded turmeric

½ teaspoon of grinded coriander

2 minced garlic cloves,

6 cups of fat-free, less-sodium chicken broth

1 (13.5-ounce) can of light coconut milk

2 ½ cups of shredded cooked chicken breast (about 1 pound)

½ cup of chopped green onions

2 tablespoons of sugar

2 tablespoons of fish sauce

½ cup of chopped fresh cilantro

4 small hot red seeded and chopped chilies, or ¼ teaspoon of crushed red pepper

7 lime wedges

Preparation
1. Boil 4 cups of water in a large saucepan.
2. Add the spinach and peas to pan then cook for 30 seconds.
3. Remove the vegetables from the pan with a slotted spoon and place it in a large bowl.
4. Add the noodles to the pan and cook 3 minutes.
5. Drain and add the noodles to the spinach mixture in the bowl.
6. Heat Canola the oil in pan over medium-high heat setting.
7. Add the shallots and the next 5 ingredients (through garlic) to pan and cook for 1 minute and stir it constantly.
8. Add chicken broth to pan, and then boil.
9. Add coconut milk to the pan and reduce the heat, and cook for 5 minutes.

10. Add the chicken, onions, sugar, and fish sauce to the pan and cook for 2 minutes.
11. Pour the chicken mixture over the noodle mixture in the bowl.
12. Add the cilantro and chilies.
13. Serve with lime wedges.

Classic Chicken Soup

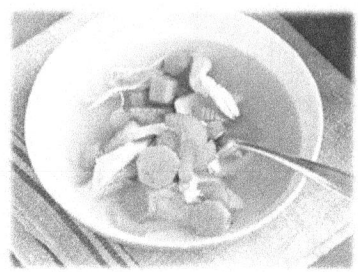

This classic chicken soup calls for chicken, sliced carrots and celery, quartered yellow onion, and is seasoned with kosher salt and whole black peppercorns.

PREP TIME: 15 mins

TOTAL TIME: 50 mins

YIELD: Serves 4

Classic Chicken Soup

Ingredients

1 3 ½ - to 4-pound chicken

6 peeled carrots

4 celery stalks

1 large quartered yellow onion

2 ½ teaspoons of kosher salt

1 teaspoon of a whole black peppercorns

Preparation

1. Rinse the chicken inside and out and pat it dry with paper towels.
2. Place the chicken in a large pot.
3. Cut 3 of the carrots and 2 of the celery stalks into 1-inch pieces.
4. Quarter the onion and add the cut vegetables to the pot with the salt, peppercorns, and enough cold water to cover (about 8 cups), then boil.
5. Reduce the heat and cook, while skimming any foam that rises to the top, until the chicken is cooked through, for about 30 minutes.
6. Transfer the chicken to a bowl and let it cool.
7. Strain the broth, discarding the vegetables.
8. Return the broth to the pot.
9. Thinly slice the remaining carrots and celery.
10. Add them to the broth and cook until soft, for about 10 minutes.
11. When the chicken is cool enough to handle, shred the meat and add it to the soup.
12. Serve into individual bowls.

Hearty Chicken Soup

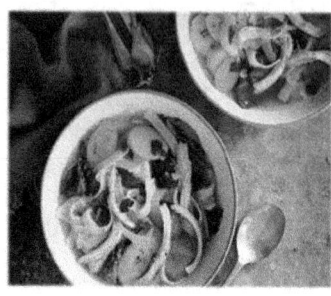

It makes sense that a classic like chicken soup would be best cooked in a classic Dutch oven. While we enjoyed the soup from all three cooking methods, the Dutch oven made the meat a little softer and juicy. The broth also cooks without a lid, so it reduces and grows richer.

PREP TIME: 25 mins

TOTAL TIME: 45 mins

YIELD: Serves 4 (serving size: 1 1/3 cups)

Hearty Chicken Soup

Ingredients

2 tablespoons of olive oil

1 ½ cups of vertically sliced onion

1 ½ cups of diagonally sliced carrot

¾ cup of diagonally sliced parsnip

3 crushed garlic cloves

7 cups of unsalted chicken stock

5 flat-leaf of parsley sprigs

3 fresh thyme sprigs

2 (6-ounce) of skinned bone-in chicken thigh

2 bay leaves

1 (1-pound) of skinned bone-in chicken breast,

4 ounces of medium egg noodles

4 cups of baby spinach

¼ cup of fresh flat-leaf parsley leaves

¾ teaspoons of salt

½ teaspoon of freshly grinded black pepper

Preparation
1. Heat a large Dutch oven over medium-HIGH heat setting.
2. Add oil to the pan and swirl to coat.
3. Add onion, carrot, parsnip, and garlic to pan and cook for 5 minutes.
4. Add the stock and the next 5 ingredients (through chicken breast), then allow it to boil.
5. Reduce heat and cook for 20 minutes or until chicken is done.
6. Remove the chicken and vegetables from the pan and let chicken stand 10 minutes.
7. Shred the chicken and Discard parsley sprigs, thyme, and bay leaves.
8. Increase heat to medium-high heat setting and add the noodles then cook for 6 minutes or until done.
9. Return the chicken and vegetables to pan and add the spinach and the remaining ingredients.

Avocado-Buttermilk Soup With Crab Salad

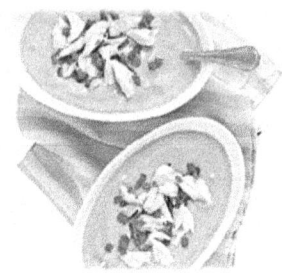

Simple orange-infused crabmeat floats atop a rich, creamy soup. If the soup seems a little too thick, add 1 to 2 tablespoons of more buttermilk.

TOTAL TIME: 18 mins

YIELD: 4 servings

Avocado-Buttermilk Soup with Crab Salad

Ingredients

¾ cup of fat-free buttermilk

½ cup of chopped fresh tomatillos

½ cup of fat-free, low heater-sodium chicken broth

3/8 teaspoons of salt

2 ripe peeled and pitted avocados

1 seeded serrano pepper

1 small garlic clove

2 tablespoons of minced red bell pepper

1 teaspoon of chopped fresh chives

1 teaspoon of fresh lemon juice

½ teaspoon of grated orange rind

Ounces of drained and shell pieces removed lump crabmeat

Preparation
1. Place first 7 ingredients in a blender and process until smooth.
2. Add bell pepper and remaining ingredients and toss gently for it to mix.
3. Spoon about ¾ cup of soup into each of 4 bowls and top each serving with about 1/3 cup of crabmeat mixture.

Italian Wedding Risotto Soup

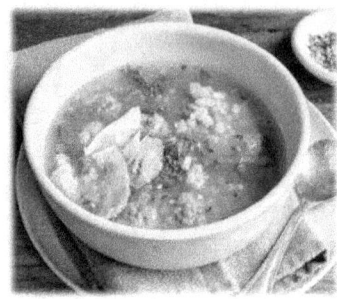

Mix up traditional Italian Wedding Soup by substituting orzo for risotto.

YIELD: Serves 4 (serving size: about 1 ½ cups)

Italian Wedding Risotto Soup

Ingredients

ounces of bulk sweet Italian sausage

1 teaspoon of Canola oil

½ cup of minced shallots

1 teaspoon of minced garlic

¼ teaspoon of crushed red pepper

cups of unsalted chicken stock

1 ½ cups of prepared risotto reserved from Sweet Onion Risotto with Cooked Kale

1 cup of chopped escarole

¼ teaspoon of kosher salt

1 ounce of shaved Parmesan cheese (about ¼ cup)

Preparation
1. Divide and shape the sausage into 26 balls (about 1 teaspoon of each).
2. Heat a large Dutch oven over medium heat setting.
3. Add the oil and swirl.
4. Add minced shallots, minced garlic, and the crushed red pepper then cook for 5 minutes.
5. Add the chicken stock and allow it to boil.
6. Add the sausage and prepared risotto reserved from Sweet Onion Risotto with Cooked Kale
7. Reduce the heat, and cook for 5 minutes.
8. Add the escarole and salt then cook for 2 minutes.
9. Divide among 4 bowls and top with shaved Parmesan cheese.

Avocado Gazpacho With Sourdough Croutons

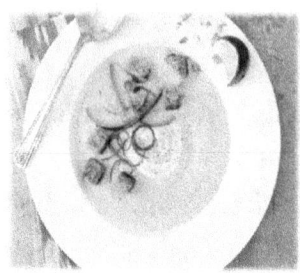

For a cool summer soup, try this avocado-flavored gazpacho made with cucumbers, sweet onion, Greek yogurt, and more.

PREP TIME: 50 mins

TOTAL TIME: 2 hours 50 mins

YIELD: Serves 4

Avocado Gazpacho with Sourdough Croutons

Ingredients

cups of chopped peeled English cucumber (about 1 ½ cucumbers)

1 cup of chopped sweet onion

1 teaspoon of olive oil

2 teaspoons of divided kosher salt

3 ripe avocados (about 1 ½ pounds)

1 cup of cold water

1 large smashed garlic clove

2 tablespoons of fresh lime juice

½ teaspoon of freshly grinded black pepper

¼ cup of plain Greek yogurt

Sourdough Croutons

Garnish: Thinly sliced green onions

Preparation
1. Add first 3 ingredients and ½ teaspoons of salt in a large saucepan over medium-low heat setting.
2. Cover and cook and stir it often for 10 minutes or until vegetables are soft. (but does not brown.)
3. Spread the mixture into a single layer on a baking sheet.
4. Refrigerate for 15 minutes or until it is thoroughly chilled.
5. Place the cucumber mixture, 2 ½ avocados, and the remaining 1 ½ teaspoons of salt in a blender.
6. Cover remaining avocado half tightly with plastic wrap in order to prevent browning.
7. Place cold water and next the 4 ingredients to the blender process until it becomes smooth.
8. Pour mixture into a bowl and cover surface with plastic wrap and chill 2 hours.
9. Thinly slice the remaining avocado half.
10. Divide gazpacho evenly among 4 soup bowls and top with avocado slices and Sourdough Croutons and garnish, if desired.

Carrot Soup With Parmesan Crisps

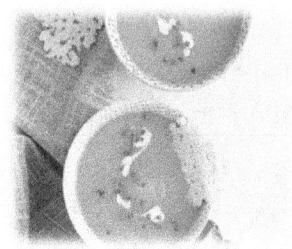

Cheese crisps are the perfect topper for this sweet carrot soup.

PREP TIME: 37 mins

TOTAL TIME: 1 hour 13 mins

YIELD: 6 - servings

Carrot Soup with Parmesan Crisps

Ingredients

1 ounce of Parmigiano-Reggiano cheese, grated (about ¼ cup)

2/3 cups of coarsely chopped carrot

2 ½ cups of unsalted chicken stock

2 cups of plus 1 teaspoon of divided water

2 cups of coarsely chopped leek, (white and light green parts only of about 2 large pieces)

1 teaspoon of white wine vinegar

¼ teaspoon of kosher salt

¼ teaspoon of pepper

1/8 teaspoon of grinded nutmeg

3 tablespoons of crème fraîche or sour cream

1 teaspoon of finely chopped fresh chives

preparation

1. Preheat oven to 350°.
2. Spread 2 teaspoons of cheese evenly into a 2-inch circle on a parchment-lined baking sheet and repeat 5 times, while leaving 1 inch between circles.
3. Bake at 350° for 8 minutes or until it turns golden.
4. Remove the pan from oven and carefully lift crisps from pan with a spatula, and place it on a wire rack.
5. The cheese crisps cool down completely.
6. Add the carrot, chicken stock, 2 cups of water, and leek in a large Dutch oven, then allow it to boil.
7. Partially cover it, reduce the heat, then cook 30 minutes.
8. Remove pan from heat, and wait 10 minutes.
9. Place half of the carrot mixture in a blender.
10. Remove center piece of blender lid (to allow steam to escape) and secure blender lid.
11. Place a clean towel over opening in blender lid (to avoid splatters). Blend until smooth.
12. Strain mixture through a sieve over a large bowl and discard the solid particles.
13. Repeat this procedure with remaining carrot mixture.
14. Add the vinegar, salt, pepper, and nutmeg.
15. Add the remaining 1 teaspoon of water, crème fraîche, and chives in a bowl.
16. Place about 1 cup soup in each of 6 bowls.
17. Top each serving with 1 teaspoon of crème fraîche mixture and 1 crisp.

White Bean And Chorizo Soup

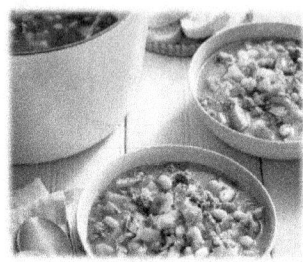

Fresh chorizo sausage gives this soup its vibrant red-orange hue and fiery flavor.

PREP TIME: **20 mins**

TOTAL TIME: **40 mins**

YIELD: Serves 6 (serving size: about 1 1/3 cups)

White Bean and Chorizo Soup

Ingredients

1-pound of fresh chorizo link sausage, with casing removed

2 tablespoons of olive oil

1 chopped large yellow onion, (about 2 cups)

2 chopped medium carrots (about 1 cup)

½ pound of small chopped red potatoes

3 minced garlic cloves

1 teaspoon of paprika

1 teaspoon of kosher salt

1 tablespoon of tomato paste

2 (15-oz.) cans of great Northern beans, drained and rinsed

1 (32-oz.) container of reduced-sodium chicken broth

½ cup of fresh chopped parsley leaves

Preparation
1. Cook the chorizo in a Dutch oven over medium-high heat setting and stir constantly, until it turns brown and get crumbled, for about 8 minutes.
2. Drain well on paper towels and Wipe Dutch oven clean.
3. Heat the oil in Dutch oven over medium-high heat setting.
4. Add onions and the next 5 ingredients, and cook until it becomes soft, for about 5 minutes.
5. Add the tomato paste, and cook for 1 minute and stir often.
6. Increase heat to high heat setting.
7. Add the beans, chicken broth, and chorizo, and then allow it to boil.
8. Reduce the heat to medium low heat setting, and cook and stir occasionally and skimming off any fat from the top, for 20 minutes.
9. Add the parsley, and serve immediately.

Two-Bean Soup With Tomato-Chive Crostini

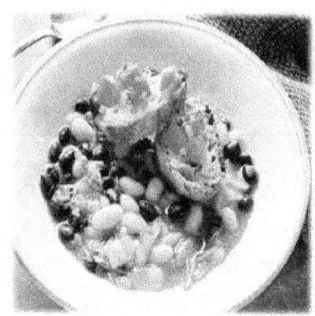

For a vegetarian version of this bean soup, substitute the chicken broth for a vegetable mushroom broth. Garnish with a tomato-chive crostino for added crunch to this 30-minute soup.

PREP TIME: 15 mins

TOTAL TIME: 30 mins

YIELD: Serves 4

Two-Bean Soup with Tomato-Chive Crostini

Ingredients

1 tablespoon of olive oil

1 cup of chopped onion

1 tablespoon of minced garlic

1 tablespoon of chopped fresh thyme

1 ½ tablespoons of white miso

4 cups of unsalted chicken stock (such as Swanson), divided

2 cups of cooked white beans, reserved from Peppered Shrimp with divided White Bean and Cauliflower Blend

¼ teaspoon of kosher salt

2 bay leaves

1 (15.5-ounce) can of unsalted black beans, rinsed and drained

2 cups of coarsely chopped fresh spinach leaves

(½ -ounce) slices whole-grain French bread baguette

Cooking spray

½ cup chopped fresh tomato

3 tablespoons of minced fresh chives

Preparation
1. Preheat the oven to 400°.
2. Heat the oil in a large Dutch oven over medium heat setting.
3. Add the onion, garlic, and thyme and cook for 6 minutes.
4. Add the miso and cook for 1 minute.
5. Add 1 cup of stock and stir until the miso dissolves.
6. Add the remaining 3 cups of stock.
7. Lightly mash 1 cup of beans and add the mashed beans, and the remaining 1 cup of beans, salt, bay leaves, and black beans to stock mixture in pan and allow it to boil.
8. Reduce heat, and cook for 15 minutes.
9. Remove pan from heat and discard bay leaves.
10. Add spinach until it is wilted.
11. Arrange the bread slices on a baking sheet coated with cooking spray. Bake at 400° for 5 minutes or until toasted.
12. Add tomato and chives in a bowl.
13. Divide the tomato mixture evenly over bread.
14. Place about 1 ½ cups of soup in each of 4 bowls and top each serving with 2 topped bread slices.

Golden Gazpacho

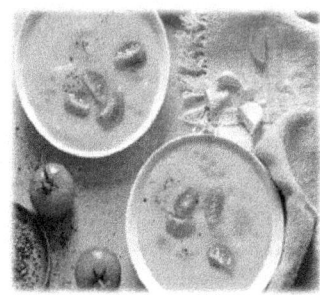

Yellow tomatoes are a little less acidic than red, making this chilled soup's flavor sublime.

PREP TIME: 25 mins

TOTAL TIME: 55 mins

YIELD: Serves 6

Golden Gazpacho

INGREDIENTS

½ cup of water

½ ounces of French bread baguette, interior crumb only, torn into small pieces

1 cup of coarsely chopped yellow bell pepper

1 cup of chopped seeded peeled cucumber

½ cup of chopped sweet onion

½ tablespoons of extra-virgin olive oil, divided

2 tablespoons of sherry vinegar

1 chopped garlic clove

2 pounds of peeled, cored, seeded, and coarsely chopped yellow heirloom tomatoes,

3/8 teaspoon of kosher salt

12 chopped red cherry tomatoes

PREPARATION

1. Add ½ cup of water and bread in a small bowl and wait 5 minutes.
2. Place the bell pepper, cucumber, onion, 3 tablespoons of oil, vinegar, garlic, and yellow tomato in a blender then process until it is smooth.
3. Add the bread mixture and salt to the blender then process for 1 minute.
4. Cover it and refrigerate for at least 30 minutes.
5. Place 1 cup of soup in each of 6 the bowls.
6. Top evenly with the remaining 1 ½ teaspoons of oil and red tomatoes.

Simple Cream Of Broccoli Soup

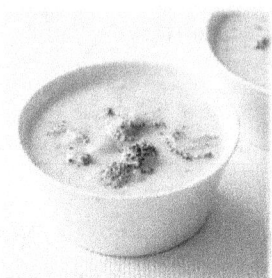

Your favorite broccoli soup recipe is easy, so you can now make it yourself! Simple Cream of Broccoli Soup is lighter than the gooey, cheesy original, but it still tastes great. The ingredients in this version really enhance the flavor of the broccoli. This is a great way to eat your veggies in an unconventional way. You can even add pasta to the soup to make it a little thicker and make it more filling. No matter how you serve it, this soup is sure to please.

COOK TIME: 25 mins

TOTAL TIME: 25 mins

YIELD: 8 servings

Simple Cream of Broccoli Soup

Ingredients

3 bags of fresh broccoli florets

1 large chopped onion

1 minced clove garlic(optional)

1 to 2 quarts of chicken broth or water

1 cup of cream or milk

Salt and pepper to taste

¼ cup of fresh chopped dill or basil

2 cups of cooked tiny pasta (optional)

Preparation
1. Rinse the broccoli florets and cover with water.
2. Add the chopped onion then cook it uncovered until broccoli is done.
3. Drain and reserve the cooking water.
4. Remove the florets and onion to a large cooking pot.
5. Add enough stock to cover.
6. You can also leave the vegetables wet, use broccoli water, and add some chicken bouillon.
7. finely chop the broccoli with a hand blender, but don't puree it.
8. Heat it well, season to taste.
9. Add the cream or milk and if extra thickening is desired then add the pasta.
10. Garnish the soup bowls with dabs of sour cream or a sprinkle of fresh herbs.
11 Serve with crackers.

Creamy Garlic Soup

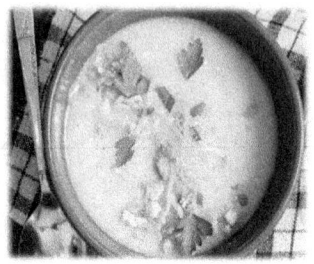

This soup is surprisingly mellow heat setting the garlic truly softens in flavor as it cooks.

PREP TIME: 20 mins

TOTAL TIME: 1 hour 20 mins

YIELD: Serves 12 (serving size: about ¾ cup of soup)

Creamy Garlic Soup

Ingredients

1 tablespoon of unsalted butter

4 cups of garlic cloves

2 cups of vertically sliced sweet onion

1 cup of cubed peeled potato

2 tablespoons of fresh thyme leaves

4 cups of unsalted chicken stock

2 cups of water

¾ teaspoon of kosher salt

1 (2-inch) strip lemon rind

1 (1-ounce) slice, cubed French bread, stale or oven-dried

¼ cup of buttermilk

1 ½ tablespoons of sherry

1/3 cup toasted breadcrumbs

2 tablespoons of grated pecorino Romano

1 tablespoon of parsley

2 teaspoons of lemon rind

Preparation
1. Melt the butter in a Dutch oven over medium-low heat setting.
2. Add the garlic cloves, onion, potato, and thyme.
3. Cover it and cook for 25 minutes and stir occasionally.
4. Add the stock, water, salt, and 2-inch strip of lemon rind and allow it to boil.
5. Cover it and cook at low heat setting for 20 minutes or until very soft.
6. Discard the rind.
7. Add the bread and stir with a wooden spoon.
8. Pour half of the soup into a blender, and remove the center piece of blender lid, to allow steam to escape and drape a clean towel over opening in lid to avoid splatters.
9. Blend until it turns smooth then pour it into a large bowl.
10. Repeat this process with the remaining soup and the return blended soup to the pan.
11. Add the buttermilk and heat over medium-high heat setting until it is very hot (do not boil).
12. Add the sherry.

13. Serve and top soup with a mixture of toasted breadcrumbs, grated pecorino Romano, parsley, and lemon rind.

Caribbean Black Bean Soup

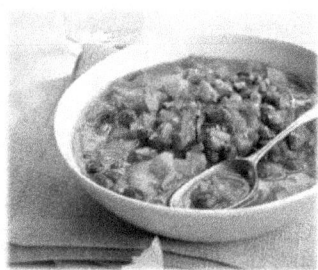

A little of this spicy soup goes a long way, so it's best when served as an appetizer soup. If you want to decrease the heat, seed the jalapeños.

YIELD: 8 servings (serving size: about 1 cup of soup, 1 tablespoon of cilantro, and 1 lime wedge)

Caribbean Black Bean Soup

Ingredients

1 tablespoon of olive oil

2 cups of chopped red onion (1 onion)

1 cup of diced green bell pepper

1 cup of diced red bell pepper

3 tablespoons of finely chopped jalapeño pepper (2 peppers)

1 whole garlic head, peeled and minced

¼ cup no-salt-added tomato paste

4 cups of organic vegetable broth, divided

1 teaspoon of dried thyme

1 teaspoon of grinded cumin

½ teaspoon of grinded ginger

½ teaspoon of grinded allspice

¼ teaspoon of grinded red pepper

1/8 teaspoon of salt

2 (15-ounce) cans no-salt-added black beans, rinsed and drained

½ cup of coconut milk

½ cup of chopped fresh cilantro

2 quartered limes

Preparation
1. Heat the large skillet over medium-high heat setting.
2. Add oil to the pan and swirl to coat.
3. Add onion and the next 3 ingredients (through jalapeño) then cook for 4 minutes.
4. Add garlic and cook 1 minute.
5. Add the tomato paste and 1 cup of broth.
6. Transfer the vegetable mixture to a 5-quart electric slow cooker.
7. Add the remaining 3 cups of broth, thyme, and the next 6 ingredients (through black beans).
8. Cover it and cook on low heat setting for 8 hours.
9. Add the coconut milk.
10. Serve the soup into bowls and top with cilantro and the lime wedges.

Vegetable-Beef Soup

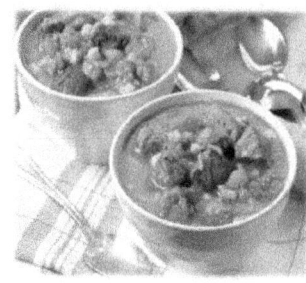

Slow-cooking top round steak with tomatoes, garlic, onion, and Worcestershire sauce creates a succulent soup full of soft beef. This soup is sure to please the whole family.

PREP TIME: 11 mins

COOK TIME: 7 hours

YIELD: 8 servings (serving size: for about 1 ¾ cups)

Vegetable-Beef Soup

Ingredients

1 ounces of all-purpose flour (about ¼ cup)

1 ½ pounds of lean top round steak, cut into 1-inch cubes

2 teaspoons of spicy herb blend

2 (16-ounce) packages of frozen gumbo vegetables mix

1 (10-ounce) package frozen of chopped onion

2 (14.5-ounce) cans of undrained diced tomatoes with garlic

2 (14.5-ounce) cans of fat-free, low heater-sodium beef broth

1 tablespoon of minced garlic

1 tablespoon of low heater-sodium Worcestershire sauce

½ teaspoon of salt

½ teaspoon of freshly grinded black pepper

Preparation
1. Place the flour in a large zip-top plastic bag and add the steak cubes.
2. Seal and shake very well to coat.
3. Remove the steak from the bag and set it aside.
4. Place a large nonstick skillet coated with cooking spray over medium-high heat setting until hot.
5. Add the steak, and cook until it is browned on all sides.
6. Place the steak and the remaining ingredients in a 4-quart electric slow cooker stir well.
7. Cover the lid and cook on high heat setting for 1 hour.
8. Reduce the heat to low heat setting and cook for 6 hours or until meat is done and vegetables are soft.

Garden Minestrone

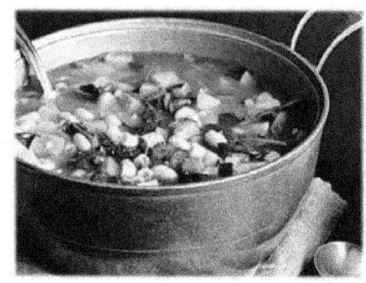

Bursting with the goodness of seven vegetables.

PREP TIME: 22 mins

COOK TIME: 58 mins

YIELD: 8 servings (serving size: 1 1/2 cups of soup and 2 tablespoons of cheese)

Garden Minestrone

Ingredients

2 teaspoons olive oil

1 cup of chopped onion

2 teaspoons of chopped fresh oregano

4 minced garlic cloves

3 cups of chopped yellow squash

3 cups of chopped zucchini

1 cup of chopped carrot

1 cup of fresh corn kernels (about 2 ears)

4 cups of chopped tomato, divided

3 (14-ounce) cans of divided fat-free, less-sodium chicken broth

1/2 cup of uncooked ditalini pasta (very short tube-shaped macaroni)

1 (15.5-ounce) can of rinsed and drained Great Northern beans,

1 (6-ounce) package of fresh baby spinach

3/4 teaspoon of salt

1/2 teaspoon of freshly grinded black pepper

1 cup (4 ounces) of grated Asiago cheese

Coarsely grinded black pepper (optional)

Preparation
1. Heat the oil in a Dutch oven over medium-high heat setting.
2. Add onion to the pan and cook for 3 minutes or until it softens.
3. Add the oregano and garlic and cook for 1 minute.
4. Add the squash, zucchini, carrot, and corn and cook for 5 minutes or until the vegetables are soft.
5. Reduce the Heat.
6. Place 3 cups of tomato and 1 can of broth in a blender and process until it is smooth.
7. Add the tomato mixture to the pan and heat up the pan.
8. Add the remaining 1 cup of tomato and remaining 2 cans of broth and boil the mixture.
9. Reduce heat, and cook for 20 minutes.
10. Add the pasta and beans to and cook for 10 minutes or until the pasta is soft and stir occasionally.
11. Reduce the Heat and Add the spinach, salt, and 1/2 teaspoon pepper.
12. Serve the soup into individual bowls and top with cheese.

13. Garnish with coarsely grinded black pepper, if desired.

Bacon-Corn Chowder With Shrimp

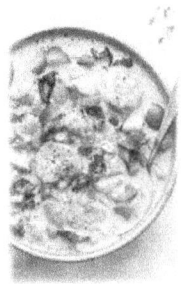

Serve this hearty chowder as either a light first course for six, or a filling main course for four.

TOTAL TIME: 20 mins

YIELD: 4 servings (serving size: about 1 2/3 cups)

Bacon-Corn Chowder with Shrimp

Ingredients

6 slices of chopped center-cut bacon

1 cup of pre-chopped onion

½ cup of pre-chopped celery

1 teaspoon of chopped fresh thyme

1 garlic of minced clove

4 cups of thawed fresh or frozen corn kernels,

2 cups of fat-free, low heater-sodium chicken broth

¾ pound of peeled and deveined medium shrimp

1/3 cup of half-and-half

¼ teaspoon of grinded black pepper

1/8 of teaspoon of salt

Preparation
1. Heat a large Dutch oven with a medium-high heat setting.
2. Add the bacon to the pan and cook for 4 minutes or until the bacon begins to get brown.
3. Remove 2 slices bacon and drain on them paper towels.
4. Add onion and the next 3 ingredients through the minced garlic then pan, and cook for 2 minutes.
5. Add the corn and cook and stir for 2 minutes.
6. Add the broth and cook it for 4 minutes.
7. Place the 2 cups of corn mixture in a blender.
8. Remove the center piece of blender lid in order to allow the steam to escape.
9. Place a clean towel over opening in the blender lid in order to avoid splatters then Blend until it get smooth.
10. Return blended corn mixture to pan.
11. Add and stir the shrimp for 2 minutes or until shrimp are done.
12. Add pepper, and salt and add half-and-half.
13. Crumble reserved the bacon over soup.

French Onion Soup

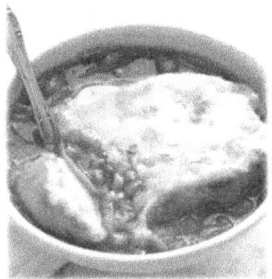

Create the delicious taste of classic French onion soup in your slow cooker. This slow cooking method allows all the flavors to meld and develop over time, creating a beautifully balanced soup. This balance of the components of the soup ensures that it's not too salty, like some other French onion soups. Plus, you will learn how to make the perfect French bread and cheese topping for the soup. This soup is truly impressive when it's finished and will wow everyone who eats it.

TOTAL TIME: 20 mins

YIELD: 4 servings (serving size: about 1 2/3 cups)

French Onion Soup

Ingredients

2 pounds of thin sliced onions

1 tablespoon of sugar

1 teaspoon of salt

¼ cup of margarine

3 tablespoons of olive oil

2 tablespoons of flour

2 cans of condensed beef broth

2 cans of condensed beef consommé

½ cup of dry white wine

1 teaspoon of Worcestershire sauce

3 soup cans of water

1 loaf of sliced French bread

Olive oil

freshly grated Parmesan cheese

freshly grated Swiss cheese

Preparation
1. Melt the margarine and olive oil together in large skillet.
2. Add the sliced onions, sugar and salt to skillet and sauté approximately 20 minutes or until it becomes golden.
3. Sprinkle the onions with flour and cook for an additional 2 to 3 minutes.
4. Add the remaining ingredients and the onion mixture to the slow cooker and cook for at least 8 hours or follow the slow cooker directions.
5. Brush 1 inch slices of French bread on both sides with olive oil.
6. Sprinkle one side with parmesan cheese and broil.
7. Put broiled side down in the soup, sprinkle the top side of bread with parmesan and top it with grated Swiss cheese.
8. Broil until it is bubbly.

Cheesy Potato Soup

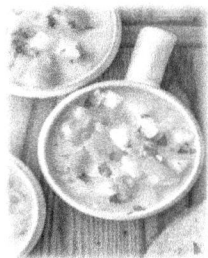

Serve a rich and hearty cheese soup with Mini Ham Sandwiches for a comforting cool-weather dinner.

TOTAL TIME: 30 mins

YIELD: 4 (serving size: 1 cup)

Cheesy Potato Soup

Ingredients

1 teaspoon of butter

1 cup of chopped onion

2 ½ tablespoons of all-purpose flour

3 cups of chopped red potato (about 1 pound)

1 ¼ cups of 1% low heat setting-fat milk

¾ cup of fat-free, LOW heater-sodium chicken broth

½ of cup water

½ cup (2 ounces) of shredded reduced-fat sharp cheddar cheese

1/8 teaspoon of grinded red pepper

2 tablespoons of chopped green onions

Preparation
1. Melt the butter in a medium saucepan over a medium-high heat setting.
2. Add onion to the pan and cook for 5 minutes or until the onion is soft.
3. Sprinkle the flour and cook for 1 minute and stir it the onion mixture constantly.
4. Add potato, milk, broth, and ½ cup water to the pan then cook.
5. Cover and reduce heat, and then cook for 10 minutes.
6. Add ½ cup of reduced-fat sharp cheddar cheese and grinded red pepper, then cook for 2 minutes or until cheese melts and stir it frequently.
7. Top each serving evenly with 1 ½ teaspoons of chopped green onions.

Slow Cooker Chicken, Bacon, And Potato Soup

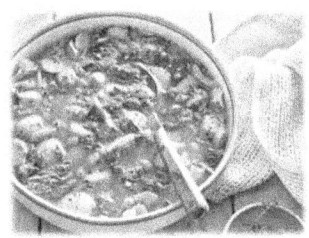

This is the most perfect soup for ushering in fall. It is hearty enough to begin the soup season. Pair with a slaw or kale side salad alongside crusty whole-grain bread for a light, satisfying dinner. This recipe is best for a weekend, when you can peep on the slow cooker after a few hours although you might not be able to leave the soup unattended to all day. It still gives the benefit of hands-free, fuss-free cooking. Either baby red, Yukon Gold, or fingerling potatoes will blend well here, because they will nicely maintain their current shape during cooking.

ACTIVE TIME: 20 mins

TOTAL TIME: 4 hours

YIELD: Serves 6 (serving size: 1 ½ cups)

Slow Cooker Chicken, Bacon, and Potato Soup

Ingredients

4 center-cut of Diced bacon slices,

1 ½ pounds of Skinned bone-in chicken thigh,

2 teaspoons of salt-free garlic-and-herb seasoning blend

2 cups of thinly sliced leek (from 2 large leeks)

1 cup of sliced carrot (from 2 large carrots)

1 cup of sliced celery (from 2 large stalks)

4 cups of unsalted chicken stock (such as Swanson), divided

¾ teaspoon of kosher salt

½ teaspoon of freshly grinded black pepper

5 thyme sprigs

12 ounces of baby potatoes

2 cups of coarsely chopped baby spinach

Preparation

1. Cook the bacon in a large skillet over medium-high heat setting until it is crispy.
2. Remove the bacon from pan, while reserving 1 teaspoon of drippings in pan.
3. Set bacon aside and sprinkle the chicken with seasoning blend.
4. Add chicken to the bacon drippings in the pan, then cook for 8 minutes, while browning on all sides.
5. Transfer the chicken using a slotted spoon to a 6-quart electric slow cooker, reserving any drippings in the pan.
6. Add the leek, carrot, and celery to the drippings in the pan and cook for 5 minutes.
7. Stir 1 cup of stock while scraping pan to loosen the browned bits.
8. Add the leek mixture of bacon and the remaining 3 cups of stock, and salt, pepper, and thyme sprigs to slow cooker.
9. Cover and cook on low heat setting for 2 hours.
10. Add the potatoes, then cover and cook on low heat setting for 2 more hours or until the potatoes gets soft.
11. Remove the chicken with a slotted spoon from the slow cooker and discard the thyme sprigs.

12. Cut the chicken into bite-size pieces and discard bones.
13. Return chicken to the slow cooker add spinach and stir until the spinach wilts.

Slow Cooker Chicken Chili

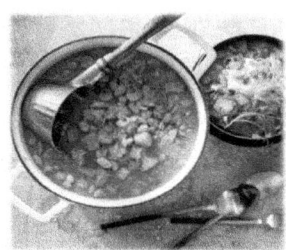

This slow cooker chicken enchilada chili recipe is a one pot meal. Enjoy the aroma as you shred the chicken, stir in corn tortillas strips, add some cheese and olives, stir, add an little more cheese and olives on top, cook for one more hour, and wow! Serve this chicken chili casserole with sour cream on top of it , and spanish rice. This is an all-time favorite recipe.

ACTIVE TIME: 20 mins

TOTAL TIME: 4 hours

YIELD: Serves 8

Slow Cooker Chicken Chili

Ingredients

3 (15-oz.) cans of rinsed, drained, and divided unsalted Cannellini beans.

1 (25-oz.) Can of rinsed and drained hominy,

3 cups of unsalted chicken stock (such as Swanson)

2 cups of peeled cubed butternut squash

1 cup of chopped yellow onion

2 tablespoons of grinded cumin

1 teaspoon of chili powder

½ teaspoon of kosher salt

2 garlic of chopped cloves.

2 oregano sprigs

1 (5-oz.) can have drained and divided diced green chilies,

1 ¼ pounds of skinless, boneless chicken thigh

½ cup of plain low heat setting-fat yogurt

6 tablespoons of divided fresh cilantro leaves,

2 ounces of pre-shredded reduced-fat cheddar cheese (about ½ cup)

¼ cup of chopped green onions

1 thinly sliced jalapeño.

Lime wedges

Preparation
1. Process 1 can of beans in a mini food processor until it gets smooth.
2. Place bean blend, remaining 2 cans beans, hominy, and the next 8 ingredients (through oregano) in a 6-quart electric slow cooker.
3. Reserve 1 teaspoon of green chilies.
4. Add remaining the green chilies to the cooker.
5. Top with chicken thigh.
6. Cover and cook on low heat setting for 8 hours.
7. Place the chicken on a cutting board and let it for cool 5 minutes.
8. Shred the chicken and add it to the chili.

9. Cover it and keep warm.
10. Process 1 reserved teaspoon of green chilies, yogurt, and 2 tablespoons of cilantro in a mini food processor until it gets smooth.
11. Place 1 ½ cups of chili in each of the 8 bowls and top evenly with yogurt mixture, remaining cilantro, cheese, green onions, and jalapeño.
12. Serve with lime wedges.

White Bean Soup

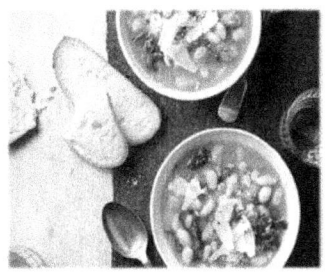

Behold! Lusciously creamy, yet cream-less. This White Bean Soup will satisfy your craving for warm, white bean soup absolutely. When the weather is cold, and you wánt to just want to stay cozy and warm, making á big pot of this Italian soup is the best thing to do. On days like these, nothing will be more comforting than this White Bean Soup. It is made with the Great Northern beans, a lot of diced hams and veggies. This Italian White Bean Soup recipe is very easy, delicious, and good for you, and it is very fast to make.

PREP TIME: 15 mins

TOTAL TIME: 8 hours 45 mins

YIELD: Serves 8 (serving size: about 1 ¼ cups of soup, 4 meatballs, and 1 ½ teaspoons of cheese)

White Bean Soup

Ingredients

6 cups of unsalted chicken stock

1 ½ cups of chopped onion

1 cup of diced carrot

1 cup of diced celery

5 chopped garlic cloves

4 fresh thyme sprigs

1 bay leaf

12 ounces of dried Great Northern beans

3 cups of stemmed and chopped kale,

2 tablespoons of unsalted tomato paste

3/8 teaspoon of kosher salt

1 pound of hot Italian sausage links, with casings removed

2 tablespoons of fresh lemon juice

1 ounce of shaved Parmesan cheese, (about ¼ cup)

Preparation
1. Place the first 8 ingredients in a 6-quart electric slow cooker.
2. Cover and cook on low heat setting for 8 hours.
3. Discard thyme and bay leaf.
4. Stir the kale, tomato paste, and salt into the bean mixture.
5. Shape sausage into 32 meatballs and arrange it on top of bean mixture.
6. Cover and cook on high heat setting for 30 minutes or until meatballs are thoroughly cooked.
7. Stir it in juice.
8. Divide the soup among 8 bowls and top with cheese.

Italian Wedding Soup

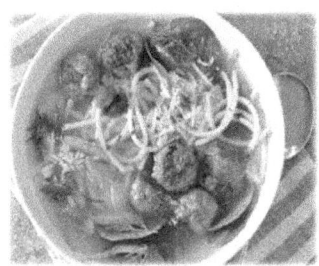

Italian Wedding Soup is a hearty, classic soup made on the stovetop! This comes together quickly for the perfect weeknight mael. And it's made with the most perfectly juicy, tender, chicken meatballs. So going for intalian Weeding Soup would be great.

YIELD: 6 servings

Italian Wedding Soup

Ingredients

12 ounces of bulk hot Italian sausage

1 teaspoon of olive oil

¾ cup of chopped onion

¾ cup of chopped carrot

2 minced garlic cloves

3 cups of unsalted chicken stock

2 cups of water

5 cups of spinach

1 ½ cups of chopped pasta mixture from Spaghetti with Anchovies, Garlic, and Red Pepper with Lemon-Caper Broccoli

¼ cup of chopped fresh dill

2 teaspoons of lemon juice

½ teaspoon of kosher salt

½ teaspoon of freshly grinded black pepper

4 tablespoons of grated Parmesan cheese

Preparation

1. Shape the sausage into 42 meatballs.
2. Heat the olive oil in a large Dutch oven over medium-high heat setting.
3. Add meatballs and cook each side for 2 minutes.
4. Remove the meatballs from the pan.
5. Add onion, carrot, and minced garlic to pan and cook for 4 minutes.
6. Add chicken stock and water and allow it to boil.
7. Add meatballs and cook for 2 minutes.
8. Stir the spinach, pasta mixture, dill, lemon juice, salt, and pepper and cook for 2 minutes.
9. Place 1 1/3 cups of soup in each of 6 bowls and top each serving with 2 teaspoons of grated Parmesan cheese.

Farmhouse Chicken Chowder

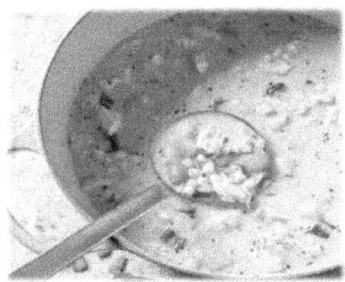

With fresh ingredients and tender, juicy chicken, this Farmhouse Chicken Chowder is just the kind of cozy dish you want to curl up with when the weather gets cool. This is a chicken soup recipe taken to the next level. With a touch of heavy cream to thicken up the broth, this recipe for chowder is rich and creamy, just the way we like it. Make a big batch for dinner tonight and then you can enjoy leftovers the rest of the week!

PREP TIME: 30 minutes

TOTAL TIME: 1 hour

YIELD: 6 servings

Farmhouse Chicken Chowder

Ingredients

1 ¼ pounds boneless chicken breast or 3 cups of cooked shredded or cut into bite-sized rotisserie chicken,

Sea salt and fresh black pepper

Flour, for dusting raw chicken

Olive oil for sautéing

1 large diced yellow onion

5 cloves of minced garlic

1 teaspoon of minced ginger, (or ¼ teaspoon grinded)

1 cup of carrot, thinly sliced into coins

½ cup of diced celery

1 teaspoon of dried thyme

1 teaspoon of dried rosemary

2 bay leaves

2 cups of parsnips, thinly sliced into coins

2 cups of cubed potatoes

2 cups of cubed sweet potatoes

1 cup of corn

5 cups of low-sodium chicken broth

1/3 cup of finely chopped fresh parsley

2 packed cups of stacked baby spinach, cut into thin ribbons (chiffonade)

1-pint of heavy cream

Preparation

Stove Top Instructions:

1. If using raw chicken, heat a few tablespoons of olive oil in a large soup or stock pot over medium heat. (for cooked chicken, skip this and go right to step 2)
2. Then cut the chicken into bite-size pieces, and season it well with salt and pepper then dust lightly with flour.
3. Cook, while turning often to make it brown on all sides.
4. Remove from pan and set it aside.
5. Add a few tablespoons of oil to the pan over Medium-low heat, sauté the onion until its cooked and translucent, add

the garlic and ginger and sauté until it is fragrant for 2 to 3 minutes.
6. Add the carrots, celery and all the seasonings.
7. Toss it well and cook for 5 minutes, while stirring often.
8. Add the parsnips, potatoes, corn, chicken broth, chicken and parsley.
9. Then cook for 30 minutes, while tasting it often and seasoning as needed.
10. Add the heavy cream to a medium size bowl and stir in 3 ladles of broth, one at a time.
11. Add the spinach to the soup and cook for 10 more minutes.
12. Remove the bay leaves before serving.
13. Slow Cooker Instructions:
14. Combine everything in a 5 or 6-quart stockpot except the heavy cream and the spinach.
15. If you are using a raw chicken, cut them in half rather than in bite-size pieces, season them well with salt and pepper and dust lightly with flour.
16. Cook for 5 to 6 hours on high heat setting or 8 hours on low heat setting while adding the heavy cream and spinach during the last hour or two.
17. Mix the heavy cream with a few ladles of hot soup before adding it to the soup.
18. Remove chicken and shred or cut into bite-size pieces, and return it back to the pot.
19. Taste and season as needed.
20. Remove the bay leaves before serving.

Lentil And KumQuat Soup

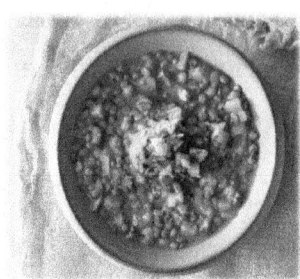

This soup has two layers of kumquats--cooked in the soup to become mellow heat setting and soft, and finely chopped with parsley for a bright topping.

TOTAL TIME: 1 hour

YIELD: Serves 5 or 6 (makes 2 qts.) (serving size: 1 ½ cups)

Lentil and Kumquat Soup

Ingredients

¾ cup (4 oz.) of chopped pancetta or bacon

1 teaspoon of olive oil

1 large finely chopped onion

¾ cup of diced carrots

¾ cup of diced celery

1 ½ tablespoons of chopped fresh thyme leaves

1 ½ cups of French green, black beluga, or regular lentils, sorted from debris and rinsed

About 6 cups of reduced-sodium chicken broth

¾ teaspoon of pepper

8 ounces' kumquats (about 24)

½ teaspoon of divided kosher salt

9 tablespoons of divided chopped flat-leaf parsley

Preparation

1) Cook the pancetta in oil, in a medium pot over medium-high heat setting until it is browned for 4 to 5 minutes.

2) Discard all but 2 tbsp. fat.

3) Add onion, carrots, celery, and thyme cook, and stir often, until vegetables start to brown for 8 to 10 minutes.

4) Add lentils, 6 cups of broth, and pepper to pot, the cover and boil.

5) Reduce the heat and cook until the lentils are almost soft, for about 25 to 30 minutes.

6) Thinly slice remaining kumquats crosswise.

7) Stir sliced kumquats into soup and add ¼ tsp. of salt.

8) Cook until the lentils are soft, for about 5 more minutes.

9) Add 3 tbsp. of parsley and a little more broth if you like.

10) Add the chopped kumquats and remaining 6 tbsp. of parsley and ¼ tsp. of salt onto bowls of soup.

Red Lentil Soup

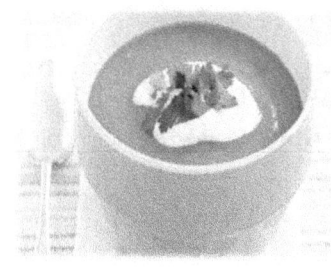

SoupCycle in Portland, Oregon, offers soups with wacky names ranging from Flemish Farm (a vegan take on French onion soup) to Who Framed Ginger Rabbit (carrot soup with ginger). Owners Jed Lazar and Shauna Lambert call this lentil soup Pot of for Goodness Sake! because the ingredients are so healthy.

ACTIVE TIME: 20 mins

TOTAL TIME: 1 hour

YIELD: 6 to 8 servings

Red Lentil Soup

Ingredients

1 ½ tablespoons of extra-virgin olive oil

1 onion, cut into ¼ -inch dice

2 minced garlic cloves

1 large celery rib, cut into ¼ -inch dice

1 large carrot, cut into ¼ -inch dice

1 (6 ounces) of baking potato, peeled and cut into 1-inch dice

1 (8 ounces) rounded cup of red lentils

1 ½ quarts vegetable stock or broth

½ teaspoon of grinded cumin

¼ teaspoon of cayenne

2 tablespoons of fresh lemon juice

Salt and freshly grinded pepper

Preparation
1. Heat the oil in a large saucepan.
2. Add the onion and garlic and cook over Moderately high heat Setting until fragrant, for about 2 minutes.
3. Add the celery and carrot and cook over Moderate heat setting for 5 minutes. Add the potato, lentils and stock, then boil.
4. Cover and cook until the vegetables are very soft, for 40 minutes.
5. Blend the soup in batches and return it to the saucepan.
6. Add the cumin, cayenne and lemon juice and season with salt and pepper.
7. Serve the soup into bowls and serve.

Potlikker Soup

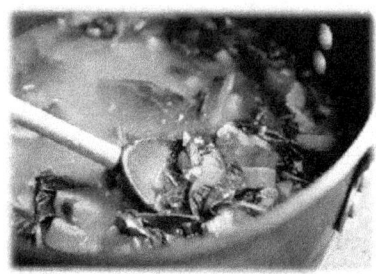

Potlikker Soup contains favorite flavors of a traditional New Year's day meal collard greens and ham hock. Serve this comforting soup with a side of cornbread.

ACTIVE TIME: 15 mins

TOTAL TIME: 6 hour 15 mins

YIELD: 6 to 8 servings

Potlikker Soup

Ingredients

1 teaspoon of olive oil

2 cups of refrigerated pre-chopped onion

½ cup of chopped carrot

2 garlic minced cloves

1 (1-pound) ham hock

4 (1-pound) packages of fresh cleaned, trimmed, and chopped collard greens

½ teaspoon of table salt

½ teaspoon of freshly grinded black pepper

¼ teaspoon of crushed red pepper

1 (32-oz.) container of chicken broth

Preparation
1. Heat oil in a large skillet over medium-high heat setting and add onion and carrot, cook for 4 minutes or until soft.
2. Add garlic and cook for 1 minute.
3. Place vegetables, 4 cups of water, ham hock, and the remaining ingredients in a 5- to 6-qt. slow cooker.
4. Cover and cook on high heat setting 1 hour.
5. Reduce the heat to low heat setting and cook for 5 hours or until ham falls off the bone.
6. Remove ham hock from slow cooker.
7. Remove the ham from its bone, chop the ham, and mix it with the soup.

Carrot-Ginger Soup

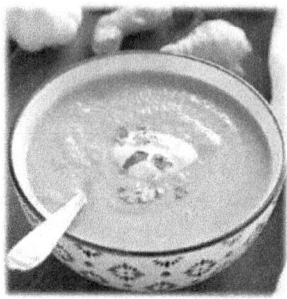

Slow-cooker Carrot-Ginger Soup provides a healthy and flavorful option for a weeknight dinner. For a refreshing summertime soup, serve it chilled.

PREP TIME: 20 mins

TOTAL TIME: 8 hour 15 mins

YIELD: 6 servings

Carrot-Ginger Soup

Ingredients

2 pounds of ends trimmed carrots (about 10 large), cut into 1-inch slices

6 white and light green parts chopped scallions

3 cloves of finely chopped garlic,

2 tablespoons of chopped fresh ginger

1 teaspoon of curry powder

2 ½ cups of LOW heat setting-sodium chicken broth

½ cup of heavy cream

Salt

Plain yogurt, (optional)

Fresh Chopped cilantro (optional)

½ pound of peeled, deveined, chopped cooked shrimp

Preparation
1. Add the carrots, scallions, garlic, ginger, curry powder, chicken broth and 2 cups of water in a slow cooker.
2. Cover and cook on low heat setting until the carrots are soft, for 7 to 8 hours.
3. Reduce the Heat and let it cool slightly.
4. Working in batches: Blend the soup in a blender and return it to the slow cooker.
5. Add heavy cream, season with salt.
6. Cover and cook until it is fully heated for, about 15 minutes or longer.
7. Serve the hot soup into bowls and top with a dollop of yogurt and a sprinkle of cilantro, if desired.
8. Place shrimp on top and serve.

Gingery Lentil Soup

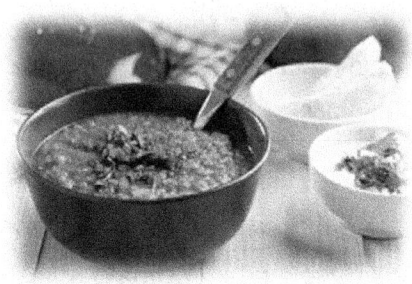

This soup recipe is sure to heal what ails you.

PREP TIME: 10 mins

TOTAL TIME: 35 mins

YIELD: Serves 4 (serving size: 1 ½ cups)

Gingery Lentil Soup

Ingredients

2 teaspoons of olive oil

3 chopped medium carrots,

1 chopped medium onion,

2 teaspoons of grated peeled fresh ginger

1 teaspoon of minced garlic

1 ½ teaspoons of curry powder

¼ teaspoons of salt

¼ teaspoon of freshly grinded black pepper

2 (14-ounce) cans of fat-free, less-sodium chicken broth, plus enough water to equal 4 cups

1 cup of rinsed and drained brown lentils

1 (14.5-ounce) can of drained and diced tomatoes

Preparation

1. Heat the oil in a large saucepan over medium heat setting.
2. Add the carrot and onion then cover and cook for 3 minutes or until softened.
3. Add the ginger and garlic and cook for 1 minute.
4. Add curry, salt, and pepper and cook for 30 seconds.
5. Add the diluted broth and lentils, then boil.
6. Reduce heat and cook for 20 to 25 minutes or until lentils are soft.
7. Add the tomatoes, then cover and cook for 5 minutes.
8. Divide soup evenly among 4 bowls and serve.

Hearty Minestrone Soup

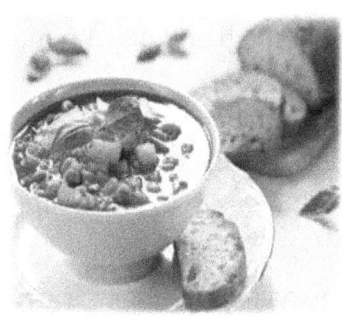

This delicious hearty minestrone soup is fat free and fully packed with vegetables full of vitamins, minerals and fiber that acts as cancer-fighters and fully support our immune system. For those looking for lentil or Italian recipes can incorporate this cooking recipes with their own favor. This hearty minestrone soup is loaded with a lot of stuffs that will make your mouth watery before it's even ready.

PREP TIME:

TOTAL TIME:

YIELD: Serves

Hearty Minestrone Soup

Ingredients

1 ¼ cups of dried white beans, soaked overnight and drained (8 ounces)

3 tablespoons of extra-virgin olive oil

2 ounces of pancetta, finely diced

2 minced shallots

2 finely diced celery ribs

1 finely diced onion

1 finely diced carrot

½ cored and diced fennel bulb

4 minced garlic

½ teaspoon of crushed red pepper

2 bay leaves

2 tablespoons of tomato paste

1 14-ounce chopped juices reserved can of plum tomatoes,

1 low heat setting-sodium chicken broth

Salt and freshly grinded pepper

1 cup of baby arugula

½ cup of flat-leaf parsley leaves

1 teaspoon of fresh lemon juice

Preparation
1. Cover the beans with 2 inches of water and then boil in a pot.
2. Cook over low heat setting until it is soft, for about 2 hours and add water to keep the beans covered.
3. Drain the beans and reserve the cooking liquid.
4. Meanwhile, in another pot, heat 2 tablespoons of the oil and add the pancetta and cook over Moderate heat setting until crisp, for 4 minutes.
5. Add the shallots, celery, onion, carrot and fennel, and cook until it softens.
6. Add the garlic, crushed pepper and bay leaves and cook, and stir, until fragrant.
7. Add the tomato paste and cook and stir it, for 2 minutes.

8. Add the tomatoes and broth, then boil.
9. Cook over low heat setting for 1 hour and add the beans and enough cooking liquid to thin out the soup.
10. Discard the bay leaves and season with salt and pepper.
11. Toss the arugula and parsley with the lemon juice and remaining 1 teaspoon of oil in a bowl.
12. Season it with salt and pepper.
13. Then Serve the soup in bowls and top with the salad.

Provencal Fish Soup

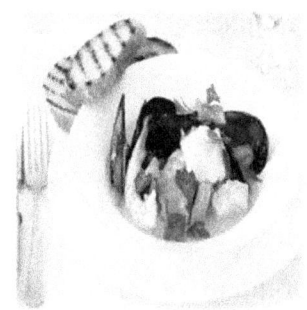

YIELD: 4 servings

If you're deciding to make dinner for a large group, it takes a courage to do that. And trying this recipe is great to start with. This is a delicious and very easy dish that will take less than halfaa an hour to make.

Provençal Fish Soup

Ingredients

¼ cup of extra-virgin olive oil

1 finely chopped onion

2 finely chopped celery ribs

1 finely chopped carrot

6 coarsely chopped garlic

4 3-inch strips of orange zest

4 thyme sprigs

2 teaspoons of fennel seeds

2 teaspoons of coriander seeds

1 pinch of saffron threads

1 teaspoon of tomato paste

1 16-ounce can of chopped and juices reserved tomatoes

2 8-ounce bottles of clam juice

¾ cup of dry red wine

½ cup of ruby port

1 ¾ pounds of coarsely chopped skinless grouper or red snapper fillets

½ pound of medium shrimp in the shell

1 teaspoon of Pernod

Salt and coarsely grinded pepper

Preparation
1. Heat the oil in a large pot.
2. Add the onion, celery and carrot and cook over Moderately High Heat Setting until softened, for 5 minutes.
3. Add the garlic, orange zest, thyme sprigs, fennel and coriander seeds and saffron and cook over Moderate heat setting and stir it until fragrant for 5 minutes.
4. Add the tomato paste and cook over high heat Setting until glossy, for 1 minute.
5. Add the tomatoes, clam juice, wine and port and then boil.
6. Add the grouper and shrimp, and partially cover it, then cook for 45 minutes.
7. Discard the zest and thyme sprigs.
8. Working in batches: Transfer the soup to a food processor and pulse until coarsely chopped.
9. Rinse out the pot and set a food mill fitted with a coarse blade over the pot.

10. run the soup through the food mill.
11. Bring the soup to a cook and add the Pernod then season with salt and pepper.
12. Serve the soup into bowls and serve.

Chicken-Vegetable Soup

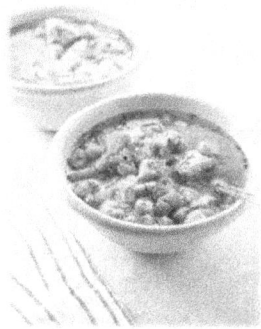

Americans of Eastern European heritage add a variety of root vegetables, such as turnips and parsnips, to chicken soup for subtle sweetness and bite. Feel free to omit them and simply add more carrot and leek, if you prefer. Be sure to cook the egg noodles separately so the starch in the noodles doesn't cloud the clear soup broth.

YIELD: 8 servings

Chicken-Vegetable Soup

Ingredients

1 (6-pound) roasted chicken

8 cups of water

2 ½ cups of chopped celery (about 4 stalks)

2 cups of thinly sliced leek (about 2 large)

1 ½ cups of (½ -inch) cubed parsnip (about 8 ounces)

1 ½ of cups of (½ -inch) cubed carrot (about 8 ounces)

1 ½ cups of (½ -inch) cubed turnip (about 8 ounces)

1 teaspoon of kosher salt

½ teaspoon of freshly grinded black pepper

1 teaspoon of chopped fresh dill (optional)

8 ounces of egg noodles

Preparation
1. Remove and discard the giblets and neck from chicken.
2. Remove and discard skin from chicken then trim excess fat.
3. Split chicken in half lengthwise and place it in a Dutch oven.
4. Cover it with 8 cups of water, then boil for 10 minutes.
5. Skim the fat from surface of broth and discard fat.
6. Add celery and the next 4 ingredients (through turnip) to a pan, and stir well, then boil.
7. Reduce the heat, and cook for 30 minutes or until vegetables are almost soft and stir it occasionally.
8. Remove chicken and wait for 10 minutes.
9. Remove chicken from the bones and shred the chicken with 2 forks to yield 6 cups of meat.
10. Discard the bones.
11. Cook the vegetable mixture for 10 minutes or until soft.
12. Return the shredded chicken to the pan.
13. Add salt, pepper, and dill, if desired.
14. Cook the noodles according to package directions, excluding salt and fat.
15. Place ½ cup of noodles in each of 8 bowls and top each serving with 1 ½ cups of chicken mixture.

Smoky Shrimp And Chicken Gumbo

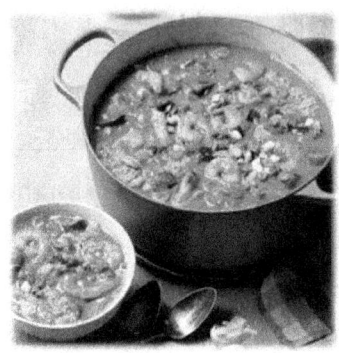

Freeze leftover stock up to three months, and use for chowder or risotto.

HANDS-ON- TIME: 58 mins

TOTAL TIME: 3 hours 13 mins

YIELD: Serves 8 (serving size: 1 cup of gumbo and ¼ cup rice)

Smoky Shrimp and Chicken Gumbo

Ingredients

Stock:

1 pound of unpeeled medium shrimp

8 cups of water

1 teaspoon of black peppercorns

4 crushed garlic cloves.

3 large chopped celery stalks,

3 bay leaves

3 coarsely chopped medium carrots.

1 coarsely chopped large onion.

Gumbo:

6 tablespoons of divided Canola oil

2.25 ounces of all-purpose flour (about ½ cup)

6 skinless, boneless chicken thigh, cut into bite-sized pieces

2 cups of finely chopped white onion

1 teaspoon of Creole seasoning

3 minced garlic cloves

2 chopped medium celery stalks

2 finely chopped medium tomatoes

1 large seeded and finely chopped green bell pepper

3 cups of fat-free, low heater-sodium chicken broth

2 bay leaves

1 cup of frozen cut okra

2 teaspoons of Worcestershire sauce

2 teaspoons of hot pepper sauce

½ teaspoon of black pepper

½ teaspoons of smoked paprika

2 cups of hot cooked brown rice

Preparation

To prepare the stock:

1. peel and devein shrimp and reserve the shells.
2. Cut each shrimp in half lengthwise and cover shrimp, then refrigerate.

3. Add 8 cups of water to the reserved shrimp shells and the next 6 ingredients (through onion) in a large Dutch oven, and then boil.
4. Reduce the heat, and cook for 1 hour.
5. Strain the mixture through a sieve into a bowl and discard solids particle.
6. Set it aside 3 cups of stock then keep it warm.
7. Reserve the remaining shrimp stock for another use.

To prepare the gumbo

1. Heat a large cast-iron skillet over low heat setting and add ¼ cup Canola oil.
2. Cook for 2 minutes, while swirling to coat pan.
3. Weigh or lightly add a spoon of flour into a dry measuring cup.
4. Gradually add flour to boil, while constantly and stir with a mix until it is smooth.
5. Increase heat to medium heat setting and cook for 8 minutes or until the flour mixture is caramel-colored and stir it frequently.
6. Cook for another 2 minutes or until mixture is chestnut-colored and stir it constantly.
7. Reduce the Heat and slowly add the warm shrimp stock, and start and stir until it is smooth.
8. Pour stock mixture into a large bowl.
9. Heat 1 teaspoon of oil in a large Dutch oven over medium heat setting.
10. Add the chicken and cook for 7 minutes while turning the chicken to brown on all sides.

11. Add the onion and the next 5 ingredients (through bell pepper) and cook for 3 minutes.
12. Return stock mixture to pan and add broth and bay leaves then boil
13. Reduce the heat, and cook for 45 minutes.
14. Add the okra and the next 3 ingredients (through black pepper) and cook for 30 minutes.
15. Add the shrimp and paprika and toss to the coat shrimp.
16. Heat a large nonstick skillet over medium-high heat setting and add the remaining tablespoon of oil to a pan then swirl to coat.
17. Add the shrimp and cook for 2 minutes or until the shrimp are done.
18. Stir the shrimp into okra mixture and discard bay leaves.
19. Serve over rice.

Corn Relish

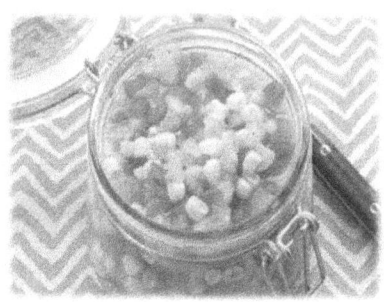

You'll need about 1 ½ pounds of butter bean pods to get 2 cups of shelled beans. You can substitute fresh lima beans.

HANDS-ON- TIME: 10 mins

TOTAL TIME: 2 hours 45 mins

YIELD: Serves 8 (serving size: ½ cup of soup and 3 tablespoons of corn mixture)

Corn Relish

INGREDIENTS

2 ½ cups of organic vegetable broth

2 cups of shelled fresh butter beans

¾ cup of chopped onion

¼ teaspoons of salt

1/8 teaspoon of black pepper

1 basil sprig

1 crushed garlic clove,

1 teaspoon of fresh lemon juice

¼ cup of fresh corn kernels

¼ cup of chopped red bell pepper

¼ cup of chopped fresh basil leaves

1 teaspoon of extra-virgin olive oil

Preparation
1. Add the first 7 ingredients in a medium saucepan over medium heat setting and allow it to boil.
2. Cover and cook for 40 minutes or until beans are soft.
3. Discard basil sprig and reserve ¼ cup beans.
4. Place remaining bean mixture in a blender add juice.
5. Remove the center piece of blender lid (to allow the steam to escape.
6. Place a clean towel over opening in blender lid (to avoid splatters).
7. Blend until smooth and let it cool down slightly, then refrigerate for 2 hours or until chilled.
8. Heat a small nonstick skillet over medium-high heat setting.
9. Add the corn and cook for 2 minutes or until browned.
10. Add the reserved ¼ cup beans, corn, red pepper, chopped basil, and oil in a small bowl.
11. Divide soup evenly among 8 bowls and top it with corn mixture.

Bbq Chicken Soup

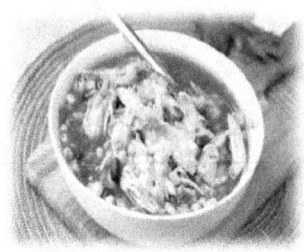

This soup is perfect for a weeknight dinner because of how speedy it is! Make this 15- Minute BBQ Chicken Soup next time you're looking for a quick recipe for dinner. It tastes similar to a BBQ chicken pizza and requires just a few simple ingredients. If you love the combination of BBQ sauce and chicken, you'll love this hearty soup. It's filled with corn and chicken, and flavored with a variety of ingredients.

HANDS-ON- TIME: 15 mins

COOK TIME: 15 mins

YIELD: Serves 4

BBQ Chicken Soup

Ingredients

2 tablespoons of extra virgin olive oil

1 tablespoon of minced garlic

1 (11-ounce) can of drained Mexican corn

1 to 2 large cooked and shredded chicken breasts

1 ½ cups of chicken broth

½ cup of BBQ sauce

½ teaspoon of kosher salt

¼ teaspoon of black pepper

¼ teaspoon of garlic salt

¼ cup fresh of chopped cilantro leaves

Preparation
1. Heat the oil in a medium pot over medium heat.
2. Add the garlic and cook, while stirring for 1 minute.
3. Add the corn and chicken breast then stir to mix.
4. Pour in the chicken broth, BBQ sauce, salt, pepper, garlic salt, and cilantro leaves
5. Reduce the heat to low and cook for 10 minutes
6. Serve it in a large bowl with a spoon and napkin! Enjoy!

Hearty Zucchini Soup

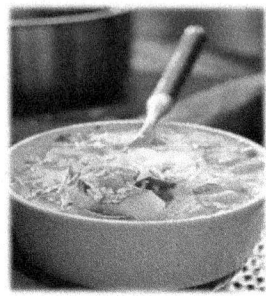

Hearty Zucchini Soup is filled with diced potato and zucchini with punches of garlic and curry flavor, making this veggie soup filling and satisfying.

YIELD: Makes 4 servings (serving size: 1 ½ cups)

Hearty Zucchini Soup

Ingredients

1 teaspoon of olive oil

1 chopped medium onion, (1 ½ cups)

2 minced garlic cloves

2 teaspoons of curry powder

1 large potato, peeled and diced

2 diced medium zucchini,

4 cups of low heat setting-sodium chicken broth

½ teaspoon of salt

¼ teaspoon of freshly grinded black pepper

Preparation
1. Heat the oil in a medium saucepan, over medium heat setting.
2. Add onion and cook for about 7-8 minutes and stir it occasionally.
3. Add garlic and curry powder then cook and stir, until fragrant for about 1 minute.
4. Add the remaining ingredients and heat to boiling.
5. Reduce the heat then cover and cook for 20 minutes.

South-Of-The-Border Beef Stew

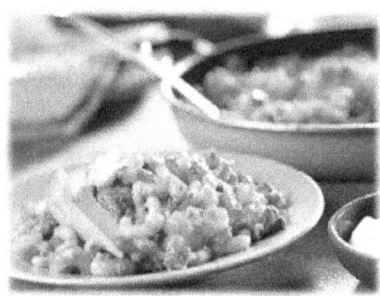

Corn and potatoes are packed in this robust stew that is good any time of year. Bring a little southwestern flavor to your dinner table with this stew. With a dash of chili powder, it has just the kick you're looking for. Plus, this fantastic recipe uses grinded beef, so it's cheaper and easier than most other beef stews. The canned soup adds flavor and a little bit of liquid consistency, while making this one of the easiest stew recipes you'll ever prepare. You are just 40 minutes away from this delicious stew!

COOK TIME: 10 mins

TOTAL TIME: 30 mins

YIELD: 6 servings

South-of-the-Border Beef Stew

Ingredients

1 ½ pounds of grinded beef

1 large chopped onion (about 1 cup)

½ teaspoon of garlic powder or 2 cloves minced garlic

1 can (10 ¾-ounce) of Campbell's Condensed Tomato Soup

1 can (10 ½-ounce) of Campbell's Condensed Beef Soup

1 cup of water

2 tablespoons of chili powder

3 medium potatoes, cut into cubes (about 3 cups)

1 (16-ounce) can have Drained whole kernel corn

Shredded Cheddar cheese, to taste

Preparation
1. Cook the beef, onion and garlic powder in a 12-inch skillet over medium-HIGH heat settings, until the beef is well browned, while stirring often to separate meat.
2. Pour out any fat and stir the soup, broth, water, chili powder and potatoes in the skillet and boil it.
3. Reduce the heat setting to low.
4. Cover and cook for 15 minutes or until the potatoes are cooked.
5. Add the corn and cook until the mixture is hot and bubbling.
6. Sprinkle it with the cheese.

Arugula Soup

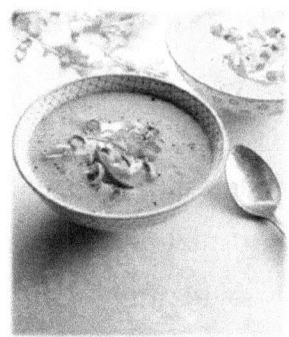

Antioxidant-rich Arugula Soup is as good cold as it is hot. And this soup is only 88 calories a cup.

YIELD: Serves 6 (serving size: 1 cup of soup with garnishes)

Arugula Soup

Ingredients

1 teaspoon of olive oil

1 medium chopped onion

2 chopped garlic cloves

1 teaspoon of cornstarch

6 cups of low heat setting-sodium chicken broth

½ cup of low heat setting-fat evaporated milk

2 (5-ounce) containers of baby arugula

¼ cup of mixed chopped herbs (such as mint, chives, parsley, and tarragon)

4 tablespoons of plain Greek yogurt

2 tablespoons of sliced chives

Preparation

1. Heat the olive oil in a large saucepan over medium low heat setting.
2. Add onion and garlic and cook until it is translucent for 5 minutes.
3. Add the cornstarch and add the chicken broth plus the evaporated milk then allow it to boil.
4. Add the arugula and the mixed chopped herbs until wilted and cover it, then set it aside for 5 minutes.
5. Use an immersion blender to blend until it is smooth.
6. Divide it among 6 bowls and garnish each with 2 tsp of plain Greek yogurt and 1 tsp sliced chives.

Colombian Chicken Soup

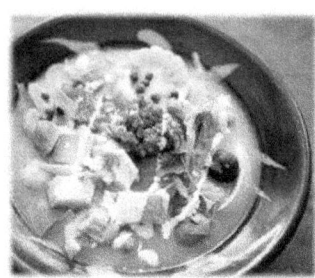

The Chicken breast in this soup adds plenty of protein but not much fat to this version of ajiaco, a cilantro-scented chicken soup that's virtually Colombia's national dish. and stir in fiber-rich brown rice turns the soup into a satisfying one-dish meal.

YIELD: Serves 6

Colombian Chicken Soup

Ingredients

2/3 cup of short-grain brown rice

1 1/3 cups of water

Salt

1 skinless chicken breast, on the bone (about 1 ½ pounds)

½ cup of thinly sliced scallions, about 3

2 smashed garlic

2 shucked ears of corn, each cut into 6 rounds

½ teaspoon of grinded cumin

½ cup plus 2 tablespoons of chopped cilantro

8 cups of LOW heat setting-sodium of chicken broth

Freshly grinded pepper

½ pound of white potatoes, peeled and cut into ¾-inch cubes

½ pound thick asparagus, cut into 1-inch lengths

1 diced Hass avocado

¼ cup plus 2 tablespoons of fat-free yogurt

1 teaspoon of drained small capers

Preparation
1. Cover the rice with the water and then boil in a small saucepan,
2. Reduce the heat and cover then let it cook until the rice is soft for 35 to 45 minutes.
3. Reduce the Heat and wait for 10 minutes, then season it with salt and fluff with a fork.
4. Meanwhile, Add the chicken, scallions, garlic, corn, cumin and ½ cup of the cilantro with the chicken broth in a large saucepan and season it with salt and pepper then boil.
5. Cook the broth over Moderately high heat Setting until the chicken is cooked, for about 12 minutes.
6. Transfer the chicken to a plate and let it cool down slightly.
7. Pull the meat off the bones and shred.
8. Strain the broth and return it to the saucepan.
9. Return the corn to the broth and discard the remaining solids particles.
10. Boil the broth and add the potatoes then cook over Moderately HIGH HEAT Setting until nearly soft, for about 8 minutes.
11. Add the asparagus and cook until the potatoes and asparagus are soft, for about 5 minutes longer.

12. Return the shredded chicken to the pot and season the soup with salt and pepper.
13. Serve the soup into bowls and garnish it with the avocado, yogurt, capers, brown rice and remaining 2 tablespoons of cilantro.

Chilled Avocado And Yogurt Soup

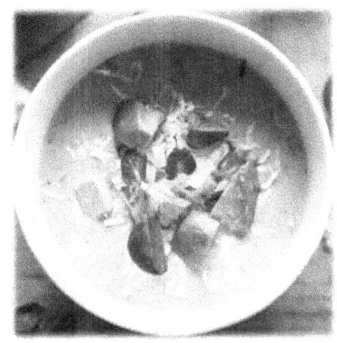

This fresh Greek-inspired soup comes together in minutes. Buttermilk gives it a soupy consistency without changing the yogurt's flavor.

PREP TIME: 20 mins

CHILL TIME: 30 mins

YIELD: Serves 4 (makes 1 qt.) (serving size: 1 cup)

Colombian Chicken Soup

Ingredients

2 large firm-ripe avocados

1 ½ cups of buttermilk

1 ½ cups of Thick and Creamy Yogurt (or store-bought plain whole-milk yogurt)

¼ cup of chopped fresh dill

2 tablespoons of coarsely chopped fresh mint, plus small mint leaves or sprigs

1 thinly sliced large garlic clove,

½ jalapeño chili, seeded

About 1 ½ tbsp. of lemon juice

About 1 tsp. of kosher or sea salt

3 radishes

Chunk of feta cheese

Preparation
1. Halve, pit, and peel the avocados and set it aside 1 half.
2. Coarsely chop the remaining avocados.
3. Whirl the buttermilk, yogurt, chopped avocados, dill, chopped mint, garlic, and Chili in a blender, until smooth.
4. Pour soup into a bowl.
5. If you'd like it thinner, add for about ¼ cup cold water.
6. Stir it in 1 ½ tbsp. of lemon juice and 1 tsp. of salt.
7. Chill until it is very cold, 30 minutes.
8. Coarsely shred radishes and cut reserved half avocado into small dice then sprinkle with a little salt and lemon juice.
9. Taste the soup and add more lemon juice or salt if you like.
10. Serve into bowls.
11. Place a tuft of radishes and a small spoonful of avocado in center of each serving.
12. Grate a little feta over soup and top with mint leaves.
13. Serve immediately (toppings will sink).

Mexican Chicken Soup

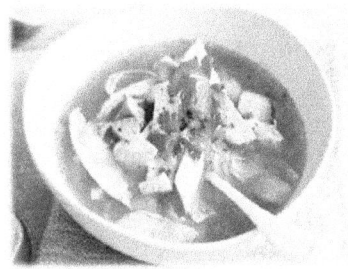

Avocado, lime and cilantro give this chicken and rice soup its Mexican flair. It makes about 8 servings and is great for when you're having a crowd.

PREP TIME: 25 mins

CHILL TIME: 1 hour 20 mins

YIELD: Makes 6 to 8 servings

Mexican Chicken Soup

Ingredients

2 whole chickens (3 ½ pounds each)

4 halved crosswise carrots

1 halved large yellow onion,

1 teaspoon of kosher salt

1 ½ cups of long-grain white rice

¼ teaspoon of black pepper

2 avocados

½ cup of fresh cilantro leaves

3 halved limes

Preparation
1. Rinse the chickens and pat dry with paper towels.
2. Place the chickens, carrots, onion, and salt in a 12-quart pot.
3. Add enough cold water (about 16 cups) to cover, then boil.
4. Reduce heat and cook gently, for 1 hour.
5. Skim off any foam that appears.
6. Transfer the chickens to plates and let it cool down.
7. Remove and discard the carrots and onion. Add the rice to the broth and cook for 20 minutes, meanwhile, shred the chicken meat, while discarding the skin and bones.
8. Add the meat and pepper to the broth and heat for 3 minutes.
9. Scoop the avocados into individual bowls and Serve the soup over the top.
10. Sprinkle it with the cilantro and squeeze on the limes. 12-quart pot is recommended.

Cucumber Gazpacho With Toasted Rye Croutons

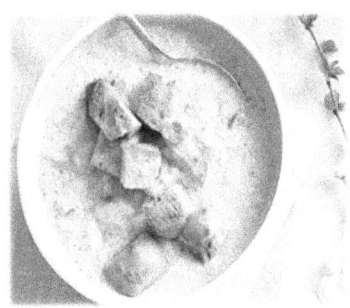

Need this soup right away? Do a rapid chill: Transfer soup to a zip-top plastic bag, and set bag in an ice bath for 30 minutes.

PREP TIME: 25 mins

CHILL TIME: 8 hour 40 mins

YIELD: Serves 6 (serving size: 2/3 cup of soup and about ¼ cup of croutons)

Cucumber Gazpacho with Toasted Rye Croutons

Ingredients

2 divided garlic cloves

3 cups of chopped peeled Kirby cucumber (about 1 pound)

2 cups of chopped green tomato (about 1 large)

1 ½ cups of chopped honeydew melon

½ cup of finely chopped sweet onion

1/3 cup of finely chopped celery

2 ½ tablespoons of red wine vinegar

2 tablespoons of chopped fresh mint

4 teaspoons of divided olive oil

1 teaspoon of chopped fresh tarragon

½ teaspoons of salt

2 seedless and cubed rye bread slices (about 2 ounces)

1 teaspoon of finely minced serrano chili

½ cup of water (optional)

Preparation
1. Finely chop 1 garlic clove and place in an 11-cup food processor.
2. Add the cucumber and the next 6 ingredients (through mint).
3. Add 1 teaspoon of oil, tarragon, and salt and process it for 1 minute or until almost smooth. (For smaller food processor bowls, work in 2 batches.)
4. Cover and chill up to 8 hours.
5. Preheat the oven to 450°.
6. Smash remaining garlic clove and place in a small bowl with remaining 1 teaspoon of oil.
7. Microwave at high heat setting for 15 seconds wait for 5 minutes.
8. Drizzle the garlic oil over the bread cubes and toss to coat.
9. Place bread on a jelly-roll pan.
10. Bake at 450° for 8 minutes or until it is browned, while turning once.
11. Stir the chili into chilled soup.
12. Add up to ½ cup of water to thin soup, if desired.
13. Serve soup into bowls and top each with croutons.

Southwest Seafood Chowder

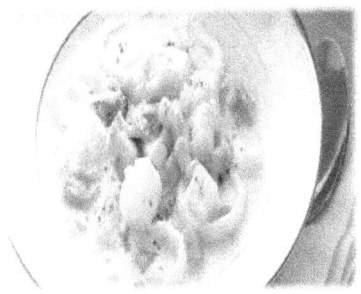

As a native New Englander, chef Steve Sicinski loves clam chowder but prefers making a healthier version with Southwestern flavors.

TOTAL TIME: 1 hour 30 mins

YIELD: 8 servings

Southwest Seafood Chowder

Ingredients

¼ cup of Canola oil

1 coarsely chopped yellow onion

5 smashed garlic cloves

2 large seeded and torn into large pieces of ancho chilies,

1 teaspoon of fennel seeds

1 cup of dry white wine

1 can of crushed tomatoes

1 cup of 2-percent milk

1 dozen of scrubbed cherrystone clams,

Salt and freshly grinded pepper

1 pound Yukon Gold potatoes, peeled and cut into ½ -inch pieces

1 finely chopped small red onion

1 finely chopped celery rib

1 finely chopped fennel bulb

1 package of frozen thawed corn kernels

1 ½ teaspoons of smoked sweet paprika

1-pound of skinless halibut fillet, cut into 1 ½ -inch cubes

1 pound of shelled and deveined medium shrimp

Oyster crackers or crusty bread, for serving

Preparation
1. Heat 2 tablespoons of the oil in a large pot.
2. Add the yellow onion, garlic, ancho chilies and fennel seeds and cook over Moderate heat setting, and stir frequently, until the onion is lightly browned, for about 8 minutes.
3. Add the wine and cook until it is reduced by half, for about 5 minutes.
4. Add the crushed tomatoes and 4 cups of water and then boil.
5. Cook over Moderate heat setting until the vegetables and anchos are very soft and the broth is slightly reduced, for about 15 minutes.
6. Add the milk.
7. Working in batches: Blend the soup in a blender.
8. Strain the soup into a heatproof bowl and rinse out the pot.
9. Add 1 cup of water to the pot along with the clams.
10. Cover and cook over high heat Setting until the clams open, for about 8 minutes.

11. Transfer the clams to a bowl and remove them from their shells.
12. Rinse to remove any grit.
13. Chop the clams and pour the clam while cooking broth into a bowl and let the grit settle, then add the broth to the soup while stopping before you reach the grit at the bottom.
14. Season the soup lightly with salt and pepper.
15. Rinse out the pot and wipe dry and add the remaining 2 tablespoons of oil to the pot and heat until shimmering.
16. Add the potatoes and cook over Moderately high heat Setting and stir it occasionally, until it is lightly browned in spots, for about 5 minutes.
17. Add the red onion, celery, chopped fennel and corn.
18. Add the paprika and cook over Moderate heat setting and stir it until the celery is crisp-soft, for about 7 minutes.
19. Add the soup and then boil.
20. Add the halibut, shrimp and chopped clams to the soup and cook until the halibut is white and the shrimp are pink, for about 5 minutes.
21. Season it with salt and pepper.
22. Serve the soup in shallow bowls with oyster crackers or crusty bread.

Lemon Grass Chicken Soup

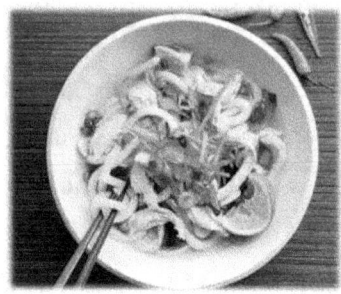

This Asian-inspired chicken soup is chock full of meat, vegetables, and delicious spices like lemongrass, ginger, garlic, and fish sauce.

YIELD: Makes 5 to 6 quarts 10 to 12 servings

Lemon Grass Chicken Soup

Ingredients

3 quarts of fat-skimmed chicken broth

2 stalks of fresh lemon grass (each 12 to 18 in. long), or 6 thin strips lemon peel (each ½ in. by 3 in. yellow part only)

12 thin (quarter-size) slices of fresh ginger

6 or 7 fresh jalapeño chilies (3 to 3 ½ oz. total)

1 ¼ pounds of cabbage

8 ounces of mushrooms

2 carrots (8 oz. total)

2 pounds of boned, skinned chicken breast halves

4 cloves of peeled and chopped garlic

1 CAN (14 ½ oz.) of diced tomatoes

About ½ cup of lemon juice

About 2 tablespoons of Asian fish sauce (nam pla or nuoc mam) or soy sauce

1/3 cup of thinly sliced green onions

5 cups of hot cooked rice

2 lemons (5 oz. each), cut into wedges

1 ½ cups of chopped fresh cilantro

Preparation

1) Boil the broth in an 8- to 10-quart pan, over high heat Setting.

2) Meanwhile, pull off and discard coarse outer layers from lemon grass and trim off and discard stem ends.

3) Rinse the lemon grass and cut each stalk into about 3-inch lengths.

4) With the flat side of a knife, lightly crush lemon grass and ginger.

5) Rinse chilies and cut one or two in half lengthwise (you can use two if you'd like it spicy), stem the remaining chilies (seed, if desired, for less heat), finely chop the stem, and reserve.

6) Add lemon grass, ginger, and halved chilies to boiling broth.

7) Reduce heat and cook, cover it for 20 to 30 minutes.

8) Meanwhile, rinse cabbage and cut into shreds about ¼ inch wide and 2 to 3 inches long.

9) Rinse mushrooms, trim off and discard stem ends and discolored parts, and slice lengthwise ¼ inch thick.

10) Peel carrots and slice ¼ inch thick.

11) Rinse chicken and cut into ¼ -inch-thick slices of either 1 ½ to 2 inches long.

12) Remove and discard lemon grass, ginger, and chilies from broth with a slotted spoon.

13) Add cabbage, mushrooms, carrots, and garlic to broth, then cover and boil over high heat Setting.

14) Reduce heat and cook until carrots are soft when pierced, 8 to 10 minutes.

15) Add chicken and tomatoes (including juice).

16) Cover and cook over high heat Setting until chicken is no longer pink in the center (cut to test), for 2 to 4 minutes.

17) Add lemon juice and fish sauce to make it tasty.

18) Serve the soup from the pan, or pour into a tureen.

19) Sprinkle with green onions.

20) Place rice, lemon wedges, cilantro, and chopped chilies in separate bowls and offer with soup to add to make it tasty.

Andouille, Crab And Oyster Gumbo

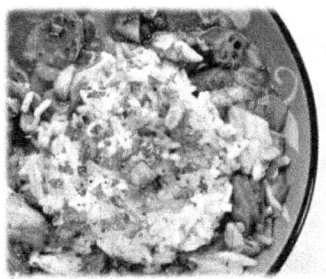

This sensational seafood-packed gumbo is terrific in its simplicity, with a foolproof roux (the mix of fat and flour that is the basis for all gumbos) that requires 15 minutes of and stir instead of the usual hour.

ACTIVE TIME: 30 minutes

TOTAL TIME: 1 hour 30 minutes

YIELD: 8 servings

Andouille, Crab and Oyster Gumbo

Ingredients

½ cup of all purpose flour

½ cup of vegetable oil

1 pound of andouille sausage, sliced ¼ inch thick

3 celery ribs, cut into ½ -inch dice

1 onion, cut into ½ -inch dice

1 red bell pepper, cut into ½ -inch dice

1 habanero chili, minced and most seeds discarded

3 minced cloves garlic

½ pound okra, sliced ¼ inch thick

2 teaspoons of dried thyme

1 bay leaf

3 tablespoons of filé powder

5 cups of chicken stock

3 cups of bottled clam juice

3 tablespoons of Worcestershire sauce

3 finely chopped (large) tomatoes

1-pound picked over lump crabmeat

24 shucked oysters and their liquor

Salt

Freshly grinded pepper

Preparation

1) Stir the flour and oil until smooth in a pot.

2) Cook over Moderate heat setting and stir it often, until the roux turns a rich brown color, for 15 minutes.

3) Add the andouille, celery, onion, bell pepper, habanero, garlic, okra, thyme, bay leaf and half of the filé powder and cook over Moderate heat setting and stir it, until the onion is translucent.

4) Add the stock, clam juice, Worcestershire and tomatoes then start boiling.

5) Reduce the heat to low heat setting and cook for 1 hour, and stir.

6) Add the remaining filé powder and add the crab, oysters and their liquor.

7) Season with salt and pepper and cook gently for 1 minute to cook the oysters.

Southwestern Chicken Soup

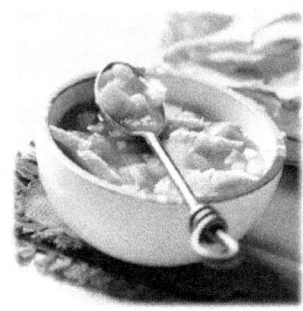

Use rotisserie chicken or leftover chicken in this easy Southwestern-flavored chicken soup.

PREP TIME: 15 minutes

TOTAL TIME: 1 hour 30 minutes

YIELD: 4 servings

Southwestern Chicken Soup

Ingredients

2-ounce of jar salsa verde

3 cups of cooked chicken pieces (1 small deli-counter rotisserie chicken or leftovers)

1 15-ounce CAN of drained cannellini beans.

3 cups of chicken broth

1 teaspoon of grinded cumin (optional)

2 chopped green onions

½ cup of sour cream

Tortilla chips (optional)

Preparation
1. Empty the salsa into a large saucepan.
2. Cook for 2 minutes over medium-HIGH heat setting, then add the chicken, beans, broth, and cumin (if desired).
3. Boil in LOW heater heat to a cook, and cook for 10 minutes and stir it occasionally.
4. Top each bowl with a sprinkling of onions, a dollop of sour cream, and some tortilla chips (if desired).
5. For a soupier dish, use 4 cups of broth.

Avgolemono Chicken Soup With Rice

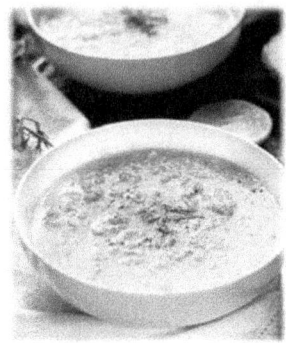

Avgolemono is a classic sauce of chicken broth, egg yolks and lemon juice the addition of a bit more chicken broth, rice and shredded chicken turns it into a satisfying soup.

YIELD: 4 servings

Avgolemono Chicken Soup with Rice

Ingredients

4 cups of homemade chicken stock or LOW heat setting-sodium broth

Salt and freshly grinded pepper

2 cups of cooked warmed white rice

2 egg yolks

¼ cup plus 2 tablespoons of fresh lemon juice

1 coarsely shredded rotisserie chicken, (1 pound)

¼ cup of chopped fresh dill

Preparation

1. Season the stock with salt and pepper in a large saucepan, and allow it to boil.
2. Transfer 1 cup of the hot stock to a blender.
3. Add ½ cup of the rice, the egg yolks and the lemon juice and then blend it until it is smooth.
4. Stir the blend into the cooking stock with the chicken and the remaining 1 ½ cups of rice and cook until thickened slightly, for 10 minutes.
5. Add the dill and serve.

Wild Rice And Mushroom Soup With Chicken

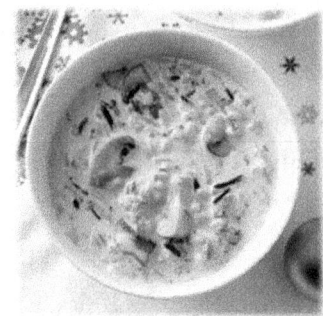

Add sliced whole wheat French bread and mixed salad greens to complete the menu.

YIELD: 4 servings (serving size: 1 ½ cups)

Wild Rice and Mushroom Soup with Chicken

Ingredients

4 cups of divided fat-free, less-sodium chicken broth

1 (2.75-ounce) package quick-cooking wild rice

1 teaspoon of olive oil

½ cup of pre-chopped onion

½ cup of chopped red bell pepper

1/3 cup of matchstick-cut carrots

1 teaspoon of bottled minced garlic

½ teaspoon of dried thyme

1 teaspoon of butter

2 (4-ounce) packages of pre-sliced exotic mushroom blend

2 cups of shredded cooked chicken breast

1/8 teaspoon of salt

1/8 teaspoon of black pepper

Preparation

1. Bring 1 1/3 cups of broth to a boil in a medium saucepan and add rice to pan.
2. Cover, and reduce heat, then cook for 5 minutes or until liquid is absorbed.
3. Heat the oil in a Dutch oven over medium-high heat setting.
4. Add the onion and the next 4 ingredients (through thyme) to pan and cook for 3 minutes and stir it occasionally.
5. Add the butter and mushrooms and cook for 3 minutes or until it is lightly browned.
6. Add the remaining 2 2/3 cups of broth, rice, chicken, salt, and pepper to pan and cook for 3 minutes or until thoroughly heated where and stir occasionally.

Carrot Soup With Brown Butter, Pecans, And Yogurt

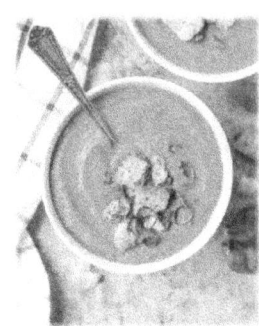

This soup brings out the natural sweetness of the carrots.

PREP TIME: 45 minutes

TOTAL TIME: **1 hour**

YIELD: 4 to 6 servings

Carrot Soup With Brown Butter, Pecans, And Yogurt

Ingredients

1 pound of carrot

4 tablespoons of divided unsalted butter

1 medium minced yellow onion

2 sprigs of fresh thyme

1 red minced jalapeño

2 tablespoons of grinded sesame seeds

1 qt. of chicken stock

Kosher salt

½ cup plus 2 Tbsp. of plain Greek yogurt

¼ cup of crushed pecans

1 teaspoon of sherry vinegar

2 tablespoons of chopped carrot tops

Maple syrup to make it tasty

Preparation
1. Peel the carrots, and cut 1 carrot into very thin rounds then reserve for garnish.
2. Cut the rest of the carrots into ½ -inch pieces.
3. Melt 2 Tbsp. of the butter in a medium saucepan over medium heat setting.
4. Add the onion, and cook and stir it occasionally, until it becomes soft for about 10 minutes.
5. Add the thyme sprigs, jalapeño, sesame, and ½ -inch cut carrots, and cook for 10 more minutes and stir it occasionally.
6. Add the stock and kosher salt to make it tasty then boil and reduce the heat.
7. Cook until the carrots are very soft for about 15 minutes
8. Reduce the Heat, and remove the thyme sprigs.
9. Blend the carrot mixture in a blender and blend till it is smooth.
10. Pour the soup back in saucepan, and add the ½ cup yogurt.
11. Ad seasoning with salt, and place the lid on the pan.

12. Melt the remaining 2 Tbsp. butter in a small cook pan over medium-high heat setting, and cook until the solids begin to brown.
13. Add the pecans, then toss and toast for about 1 minute.
14. Reduce the Heat, and add the vinegar.
15. Serve the soup in bowls and Dollop each serving with the remaining yogurt and the pecan brown butter.
16. Sprinkle with carrot coins and carrot tops, and finish with a drizzle of maple syrup.

Chard And White Bean Soup

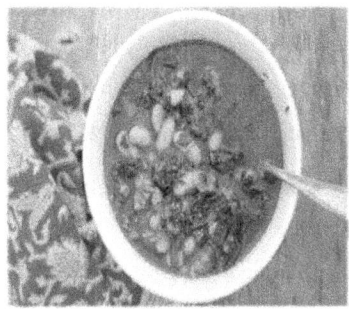

While the soup cooks, brush some slices of country bread or levain with olive oil and toast them, to serve with the hot soup.

YIELD: Makes 2 ½ quarts 4 to 6 servings

Chard and White Bean Soup

Ingredients

1 bunch of Swiss chard (about 1 lb.)

1 teaspoon of olive oil

1 teaspoon of minced garlic

1-quart of fat-skimmed chicken broth

2 cans (15 oz. each) of drained and rinsed Cannellini beans,

About ½ cup of fresh-grated parmesan cheese

Salt and fresh-grinded pepper

Preparation

1. Rinse the chard well, trim off and discard the discolored stem ends.

2. Tear the leaves from stems and thinly slice the stems crosswise and cut the leaves into 1-inch pieces.
3. Add the oil into a 4- to 5-quart pan over medium heat setting.
4. Add the chard stems and garlic and stir often until stems are limp for about 10 minutes.
5. Add the chard leaves and broth, then add 3 cups of water.
6. And allow it to boil and stir occasionally, until the chard is soft for 10 minutes.
7. Add the beans and stir occasionally until hot, for 1 to 2 minutes.
8. Add ½ cup of parmesan cheese, salt and pepper to make it tasty.
9. Serve into bowls and add more parmesan.

Baked Potato And Bacon Soup

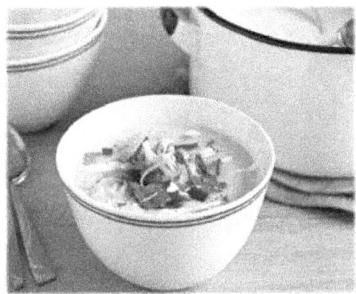

This warm and comforting potato and bacon soup is a delicious choice for a crisp fall evening. This kid-friendly soup is also gluten-free.

YIELD: 9 cups of (serving size: 1 cup of soup, about 1 teaspoon of bacon, about 1 teaspoon of cheese, and about 1 teaspoon of green onions)

Baked Potato and Bacon Soup

Ingredients

2 ½ pounds of baking potatoes

bacon slices

2 ¼ cups of chopped onion

½ teaspoons of salt

3 minced garlic cloves

1 bay leaf

3 ¾ cups of 1% low heat setting-fat milk

½ teaspoon of black pepper

1 ½ cups of fat-free, low heater-sodium chicken broth

2 tablespoons of chopped fresh parsley (optional)

½ cup of sliced green onions

½ cup (2 ½ ounces) of finely shredded reduced-fat sharp cheddar cheese

Preparation
1. Preheat oven to 400°.
2. Pierce potatoes with a fork and bake at 400° for 1 hour or until soft.
3. Let it cool down slightly.
4. Partially mash the potatoes, including skins, with a potato masher and set it aside.
5. Cook bacon in a Dutch oven over medium heat setting until crisp.
6. Remove bacon from the pan and crumble.
7. Add onion to the bacon drippings in the pan and cook for minutes.
8. Add salt, garlic, and bay leaf and cook 2 minutes.
9. Add potato, milk, pepper, and broth then boil.
10. Reduce the heat, and cook for 10 minutes.
11. Discard the bay leaf.
12. Top individual servings with bacon, green onions, and cheese.

Amish Chicken Soup

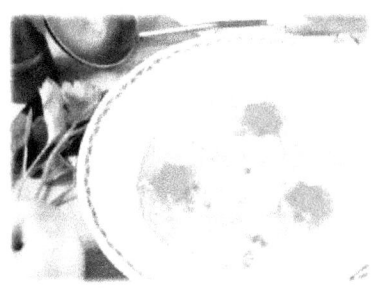

A hot bowl of chicken noodle soup is always comforting and delicious. This Amish Chicken Soup is a classic homemade chicken soup recipe that uses egg noodles, which are found in many Amish dishes. Making this chicken soup from scratch means the broth is full of savory flavor and the variety of vegetables will remind you of the chicken soup you've loved since you were a kid. This soup is easy to make, so you'll want it in your recipe box for good.

PREP TIME: 15 mins

COOK TIME: 3 hours

Amish Chicken Soup

Ingredients

3 pounds of chicken

2 quarts of water

1 ½ cup of chicken stock

2 cups of chopped carrots

2 cups of chopped celery

1 cup of chopped onions

1 tart of chopped apple

2 teaspoons of salt

Pepper to taste

4 cups of egg noodles

Preparation
1. Put the chicken in a large pot of water.
2. Cover and cook about 2 ½ hours, or until chicken is soft.
3. Remove the chicken from the pot and strain the broth.
4. Separate the bone from the chicken and return it to the pot together with the strained broth
5. Add the chicken, stock, carrots, celery, onions, apple, salt, and pepper and cook until the vegetables are soft.
6. Add the noodles and cook for another 8 to 10 minutes.
7. Then Serve hot.

Conclusion

Eating soups is a convenient way to share great times with our loved ones, experience other cultures through the flavors of their cuisines, and improve our culinary knowledge and skills. Their varieties all over the world like a delicate bowl of broth with a wonderful smell of ginger, a rich chili recipes! This book covers over 100 soup recipes. It will also help you come up with your own unique recipes. Soup recipes are certainly forgiving dishes. Whatever dish you'll make will surely be appreciated by your loved ones.

Part 2

Fish Chowder

Any milk white fish will work, cod is the easiest to find but can be substituted with something a bit more flavorful. The soup will be better if it rests 30 minutes before serving.

Preparation Time: **15 minutes**

Total Cooking Time: **45 minutes**

Serving Size: **6**

Ingredient List:

- 4 slices of bacon
- 2 onions
- 3 potatoes
- 2 ½ cups fish stock
- 1 bay leaf
- 1 tbsp. fresh thyme
- 1 ½ tsp. salt
- ¼ tsp. pepper
- 1 ½ to 2 lbs. cod fillets or other firm white fish
- 1 ½ cups heavy cream

Directions:

Mince onions, and peel and cut the potatoes into ¾ inch cubes.

Dice the bacon and put it in a pot over medium heat and cook until it has rendered its fat.

Add in the onions and cook until they are golden and translucent.

Add the potatoes, bay, thyme, stock, salt and pepper and cook until the potatoes are more or less done, about 10-15 minutes.

Make sure the fish is completely without bones and skin then cut it into 1 inch cubes.

Add the cream and the fish to the soup and reduce heat to low. Cook another 10 minutes, stirring frequently.

Cream Of Black Carrots With Spinach Pesto And Toasted Pine Nuts

The best red wine is merlot but any fruity full-bodied red wine will work. The longer it sits the better. Two hours is the minimum but if it can sit for 24 hours before serving it's better.

Preparation Time: **20 minutes**

Cook time 20 minutes

Serving Size: **4**

Ingredient List:

- 1 pound of black carrots
- 1 cup of fresh baby spinach
- 3 Tbsp. freshly grated parmesan
- 4 Tbsp. pine nuts + 4 Tbsp. toasted pine nuts
- 1 onion
- 1 clove garlic
- 4 Tbsp. basmati rice
- 4 cups water
- 7-8 Tbsp. extra-virgin olive oil
- Salt

Directions:

Peel and dice the carrots.

Mince the onion.

Toast half of the pine nuts in a pan.

Heat 2 Tbsp. of oil in a pot over medium heat and add in the onions and cook until golden.

Add in the carrots, the rice and the water.

Cover and let cook until the carrots are soft and the rice is cooked about 20 minutes.

In the meantime, put the spinach, 4 Tbsp. of pine nuts, the parmesan, the pressed garlic, a pinch of salt and the rest of the oil in the blend and blend until smooth.

When the soup is ready, blend until completely smooth.

Serve the soup in a bowl with the spinach pesto amply drizzled on top and the toasted pine nuts sprinkled on top.

Lentil Soup

The best lentils are French green lentils but regular green lentils as well as black or brown ones are fine too. Using smaller red lentils or large lentils will vary the cooking time.

Preparation Time: **10 minutes**

Waiting time: 8 hours minimum

Total Cooking Time: **60 minutes**

Serving Size: **4**

Ingredient List:

- 3 slices bacon
- 1 onion
- 2 carrots
- 3 cloves garlic
- 1 potato
- 1 bay leaf
- ½ tsp. thyme
- 1 cup lentils
- 1 tsp. salt
- ½ cup dry white wine
- 4 cups chicken broth
- 2 cups water
- 4 Tbsp. high quality extra virgin oil (to pour on top before serving)

Directions:

Put the lentils in water the night before or the morning of, letting them soak at least 8 hours.

Right before cooking them, drain the water and rinse them, picking out any stones or bad lentils.

Chop the bacon and put it over low heat in a dutch oven or large pot.

In the meantime, dice the onion, peel and dice the carrot and peel and chop the potato.

When the bacon pieces are crispy and have rendered all their fat, raise the heat to medium and add the onion and carrot.

Cook until the onion is golden, and then add the pressed garlic.

When the garlic becomes fragrant, add the lentils and stir for a few minutes, then add the wine and stir until it as all evaporated.

Add in the thyme and bay, the potato, broth and water.

Cook over medium high heat for about 35 minutes, until the lentils are soft but not mushy.

Shrimp Bisque

The shrimp shells contribute a huge amount of flavor to the broth and this step shouldn't be skipped.

Preparation Time: **20 minutes**

Total Cooking Time: **30 minutes**

Serving Size: **4-6**

Ingredient List:

- 2 pounds shell-on shrimp
- 6 Tbsp. butter
- 1 carrot
- 1 rib celery
- 1 onion
- 1 clove garlic
- 3 Tbsp. flour
- 2 cups wine
- 4 cups clam juice or seafood stock
- 1 14 ½ ounce can diced tomatoes
- 1 sprig fresh tarragon
- 1 cup heavy cream
- 1 Tbsp. lemon juice
- pinch cayenne pepper
- Salt and pepper

Directions:

Peel the shrimp and set aside.

In a pot heat two Tbsp. of butter and add in the shells of the shrimp and cook for a few minutes then pour about 3 Tbsp. of wine and cook until evaporated.

Then add in the clam juice or seafood broth.

Mince the onion and celery, peel and mince the carrot.

Heat the rest of the butter in a large pot and add in the onions, carrots and celery, cooking for about 10 minutes.

Press in the garlic and cook until fragrant, about 30 seconds.

Sift in the flour and stir until it has coated the vegetables and there are no traces.

Slowly pour in the wine, turn up the heat and cook until the wine as evaporated.

Stir in the tomatoes, tarragon and strain in the stock, and then bring to a boil.

Cover and low the heat to low, stirring frequently for about 20 minutes.

Take out the tarragon and blend until completely smooth, return to pot and add the cream.

Over medium heat, stirring constantly, add the lemon juice, cayenne and shrimp, cook for a few minutes.

Taste and adjust salt and pepper if needed.

Lentil Soup With Sausage

The best lentils are French green lentils but regular green lentils as well as black or brown ones are fine too. Using smaller red lentils or large lentils will vary the cooking time. The sausage should be fairly heavily spiced but the degree of spiciness can be changed according to taste. The tomato and the carrots work together with the spiciness so it can be considerably spicy but still work well in the soup without burning everyone's mouth. To decrease spiciness even more while still leaving the flavor, just add a potato.

Preparation Time: **15 minutes**

Waiting time: 8 hours minimum

Total Cooking Time: **65 minutes**

Serving Size: **4-6**

Ingredient List:

- 2 cups lentils
- 1 pound spicy sausage like luganega, chorizo or andouille
- 1 onion
- 3 carrots
- 5 cups water
- 2 cups chicken broth
- 2 bay leaves
- 3 cloves garlic
- 1 14 ½ ounce can diced tomatoes
- 5 Tbsp. extra-virgin olive oil

Directions:

Put the lentils in water the night before or the morning of, letting them soak at least 8 hours.

Right before cooking them, drain the water and rinse them, picking out any stones or bad lentils.

Dice an onion and peel and dice the carrots.

Take the sausage and squeeze it out of its containing intestines and break it up into small pieces.

Put the pieces into a large pot over medium heat until the sausage is cooked and there is a good amount of fat in the pot.

Put the onions and carrots in the pot with the now cooked sausage and cook until the onions are golden.

Add in the pressed garlic, bay leaves and diced tomatoes and their juices.

Stir well and bring to a boil then the lentils, broth and water.

Cook over medium heat for about 35 minutes stirring when needed until the lentils are soft but not mushy.

Cream Of Spinach Soup

The spinach should be fresh baby spinach as regular spinach won't be as good. Frozen spinach can work in a pinch. The eggs should be as fresh as possible. The cream shouldn't be substituted with milk. It will not be thick enough and it will lack flavor.

Preparation Time: **10 minutes**

Total Cooking Time: **40 minutes**

Serving Size: **4**

Ingredient List:

- 1 pound fresh baby spinach
- 1 onion
- 2 potatoes
- 3 Tbsp. butter
- 1 Tbsp. flour
- 4 cups vegetable broth
- ½ cup heavy cream
- ½ baguette
- Salt and pepper
- 4 eggs

Directions:

Mince the onion and peel and cut the potatoes into small cubes. In a pot melt the butter over medium heat and add the onions. When the onions are golden and translucent, sift in the flour and stir until it completely coats the onions and absorbs the butter.

Slowly pour in the broth and bring to a boil.

Add in the potato and cook until the potatoes are soft.

Add in the spinach and cook for about 5 minutes.

Blend the soup completely until smooth and return to pot.

Add in the cream and reduce the heat to low.

Break the egg directly onto the soup being carefully not to break the yolk, cover and cook for about 3 minutes until the white is solid but the yolk is runny.

Slice the baguette into ½ inch slices and toast then serve with the soup.

Split Pea Soup With Ham

The ham is optional but is a great additive to the soup both nutritionally and flavor wise.

Preparation Time: **10 minutes**

Total Cooking Time: **1 hour 20 minutes**

Serving Size: **4-6**

Ingredient List:

- 3 Tbsp. butter
- 1 onion
- 2 cloves garlic
- 5 cups water
- 2 cups chicken stock
- 1 pound ham steak
- 1 pound green split peas (about 2 cups)
- 2 bay leaves
- 2 carrots
- 1 celery rib
- Salt and pepper

Directions:

Mince the onions and cut the ham into cubes. Peel and slice the carrot thinly, and dice the celery.

Heat the butter in a large pot or dutch oven over medium heat and when it is completely melted, add the onion, carrots and celery, cooking until the onion is golden and translucent.

Add the garlic and cook until fragrant.

Add the lentils, water, stock and bay leaves cover and cook over low heat for about an hour and a half, stir occasionally.

Add the cubes of ham into the soup and cook until the peas have mostly lost their form, about 45-60 minutes more.

Egg Flower Soup

The eggs should be as fresh as possible. A great addition is tofu. It takes on the flavor of the soup and it adds a nice texture. It should be firm tofu and added right after the eggs.

Preparation Time: **5 minutes**

Total Cooking Time: **10 minutes**

Serving Size: **2**

Ingredient List:

- 4 cups chicken stock
- ½ tsp. sesame oil
- ½ tsp. salt
- Pinch of sugar
- Pinch white pepper
- ¼ cup cornstarch
- ½ cup water
- 3 eggs
- 1 scallion

Directions:

In a large pot bring the broth to a boil.

Mix the water and the cornstarch.

Add in the salt, sugar, pepper and the cornstarch mix.

Boil for 5 minutes.

In another bowl, beat the eggs.

Stir the broth in one direction so that the broth continues to swirl then start to slowly drizzle in the egg that it forms ribbons.

Slice the scallion at an angle and put on the soup off heat.

Tortilla Soup

Flour tortillas won't come out as well as corn tortillas. The suggested toppings are lime, Hass avocado, fresh cilantro leaves, crumbled cotija cheese, or diced Monterey Jack cheese and sour cream.

Preparation Time: **15 minutes**

Total Cooking Time: **40 minutes**

Serving Size: 4-6 as an appetizer

Ingredient List:

- 8 corn tortillas
- 3 Tbsp. vegetable oil
- 2 chicken breasts
- 8 cups chicken broth
- 2 onions
- 4 cloves garlic
- 8 sprigs fresh cilantro
- 1 sprig fresh oregano
- 2 tomatoes
- 1 jalapeño
- 1 chipotle chili adobo and 1 Tbsp. adobo sauce
- Salt

Directions:

Preheat the oven to 400 F.

Coat the corn tortillas in vegetable oil and sprinkle with salt and cut into eighths.

Arrange wedges on a cookie sheets so that they don't overlap and bake until golden brown and crispy, about 8-13 minutes.

Finely dice the onions and the chipotle, and chop the tomatoes.

Remove the skin, fat, and bones from the chicken breasts.

Heat the broth in medium large pot over medium heat and add ½ an onion, 2 cloves of garlic and ½ of the cilantro and oregano.

Cook about 15 minutes or until the chicken breasts are cooked through.

Remove the chicken and set it aside.

Filter the broth.

Puree the remaining onion, cilantro, oregano and garlic, the jalapeño, the tomatoes, the chipotle and the adobo sauce.

Add directly to the now empty pot and cook until darkened, about 10 minutes.

Add the filtered broth back in and cook for about 15 minutes.

Add more salt or adobo, according to taste.

Shred the chicken and add in the soup that has been taken of the heat.

Put the baked tortilla wedges in each bowl and ladle the soup over them, then add preferred garnishes.

Pork Ramen

The pork can be substituted for other cuts but it should they should have the same fat content and tenderness. The ramen can be bought at an important store or just a cheap store bought ramen with the seasoning pack discard. The ramen should only be made when the pork is ready because it will get gummy if it sits.

Preparation Time: **20 minutes**

Total Cooking Time: **50 minutes**

Serving Size: **4**

Ingredient List:

- 1 pounds boneless pork ribs
- ½ ground pork
- 1 Tbsp. vegetable oil
- 1 onion
- 6 cloves garlic
- 1 1-inch piece ginger
- 8 cups chicken broth
- 4 3oz packages ramen noodles
- 3 Tbsp. red miso
- 2 Tbsp. soy sauce
- 1 Tbsp. mirin
- ½ tsp. toasted sesame oil
- 2 scallions
- 1 Tbsp. sesame seeds

Directions:

Cut the pork ribs into 1/8 inch slices.

Peel and smash the garlic and peel the ginger and cut it into ¼ inch slices.

Mince the onion.

Heat the oil in a large pot or dutch oven over medium heat and add in the ground pork and cook for about 10 minutes.

Add in the onion, garlic and ginger and cook for about 2 minutes,

Add the broth, cover, lower heat and cook for about 30 minutes.

Strain broth and discard the solids.

In a pot with water and salt, boil the ramen noodles for about 2 minutes then strain.

In a clean pot, add in the soy sauce, mirin, sesame oil, strained broth and the sliced pork.

Cook for about 3-4 minutes.

Off heat, add in the miso, sliced scallions and sesame seeds.

Portion the noodles into the bowls and ladle the soup over them.

Minestrone

This recipe is quite versatile. A variety of vegetables can be added or taken about according to taste. If pasta is added, a pinch more salt and a bit more water should be added.

Preparation Time: **25 minutes**

Total Cooking Time: **90 minutes**

Serving Size: 4-6 as an appetizer

Ingredient List:
- 2 large potatoes
- 2 cups of cooked pinto beans
- 1 tomato
- 2 carrots
- ½ cup frozen peas
- 1 celery rib
- 1 bay leaf
- ½ cup green beans
- 1 clove garlic
- 5 cups chicken broth
- 1 onion
- 1 leek (white part only)
- 1 zucchini
- 3 slices of bacon
- 1 cup of squash cubes
- 1/3 head shredded cabbage
- ¼ tsp. red pepper flakes

- Salt
- Parmesan
- Extra-virgin olive oil
- Optional: 2 ounces of very short pasta like dittalini can be added in the last 5 minutes of cooking

Directions:

Peel and cut the potatoes and tomatoes into 1 inch cubes, peel and thinly slice the carrots, prepare the green beans, dice the onions and leek, half and slice the zucchini, cube the squash and shred the cabbage and chop the bacon.

Cook the bacon in a large pot over medium heat until it is crispy and has rendered all its fat.

Add the onions, carrots, celery and leeks into the pot with the bacon and cook until the onions are golden and translucent.

Add all the rest of the ingredients except the parmesan and oil and cook until all the vegetables are soft about 25-35 minutes.

When the vegetables are cooked, take it off the heat and add a few Tbsp. of parmesan and drizzle some extra virgin olive oil on top before serving.

Potato Wakame Miso Soup

Wakame is a type of seaweed that can be found wherever the kombu and katsuobushi are found. Most supermarkets have all these ingredients as well as the miso paste in the important section. Miso comes in various shades, the lightest (golden) being the least strong and the darkest the strongest.

Preparation Time: **5 minutes**

Total Cooking Time: **40 minutes**

Serving Size: **2**

Ingredient List:

- ½ ounce kombu
- ½ ounce katsuobushi
- 4 1/3 cups water
- 1 potato
- 2-3 Tbsp. of dried wakame, or 4-5 Tbsp. fresh wakame
- 3-4 Tbsp. lightly colored miso

Directions:

Put the water, kombu and katsuobushi in a pot and bring to a boil over medium heat then lower the heat to low and cook for about 25 minutes.

Peel the potato and cut into ½ cubes.

Strain the broth and throw out the kombu and katsuobushi.

The broth, called dashi, should be lightly colored.

Clean out the pot and return the dashi and bring it to a boil.

Add in the potato and cook until tender.

Add in the dried wakame and cook for another 5 minutes. Off heat add in the miso.

Black Bean Soup

To save a lot of time, it is possible to use canned beans, but a lot of flavor is lost. Suggested garnishes are limes, minced cilantro leaves, finely diced red onion, diced avocado, and sour cream.

Preparation Time: **15 minutes**

Total Cooking Time: **2.5 hours**

Serving Size: **2-3**

Ingredient List:

- 1 cups dried black beans
- 2 oz. ham
- 1 bay leaf
- 3 cups water
- ⅛ tsp. baking soda
- 1 tsp. salt
- 2 Tbsp. olive oil
- 1 onion
- ½ carrot
- 1 ribs celery
- 3 cloves garlic
- ½ tsp. red pepper flakes
- ½ Tbsp. ground cumin
- 3 cups chicken broth
- 1 Tbsp. lime juice

Directions:

Put the beans, ham, bay leaf, water and baking soda in a large pot or dutch oven with a tight lid and boil over medium heat for about 75-90 minutes, remove the scum as it comes up and stir occasionally.

Take the ham out (which will be dark due to the color of the beans) and cut it into cubes, and then set it aside.

Take out the bay leaf but don't drain the beans.

While the beans are cooking mince the onion, peel and dice the carrot, and dice the celery.

Heat the oil in another large pot or dutch oven and add in the onions, carrots and celery, and cook until the onions are golden and translucent.

Add in the garlic, the cumin and pepper flakes and cook until fragrant then add the beans their cooking liquid and the broth and boil, then reduce the heat to low and cook uncovered for about 30 minutes.

For a creamier denser soup, take about 1 cup and blend it until smooth and then add back in and then bring it to a boil again.

Off heat add the ham back in and serve with desired garnishes.

www.ingramcontent.com/pod-product-compliance
Lightning Source LLC
Chambersburg PA
CBHW071438070526
44578CB00001B/135